Contents

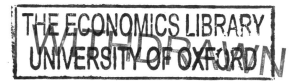
INTENSIFYING ACTION
AGAINST
HIV/AIDS in AFRICA
Responding to a Development Crisis

AFRICA REGION
THE WORLD BANK

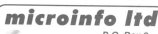

microinfo ltd

P.O. Box 3
Omega Park
Alton
Hampshire
GU34 2PG
United Kingdom

Tel: 01420 86848   Fax: 01420 89889
e-mail: ops@microinfo.co.uk
URL: http://www.microinfo.co.uk/

Library of Congress Cataloging-in-Publication Data has been applied for.

Foreword

HIV/AIDS has spread with ferocious speed. Nearly 34 million people in the world are currently living with HIV/AIDS, one-third of whom are young people between the ages of 10 and 24. The epidemic continues to grow, as 16,000 people worldwide become newly infected each day. AIDS already accounts for 9 percent of adult deaths from infectious disease in the developing world, a share that is expected to quadruple by 2020.

Nowhere has the impact of HIV/AIDS been more severe than Sub-Saharan Africa. All but unknown a generation ago, today it poses the foremost threat to development in the region. By any measure, and at all levels, its impact is simply staggering:

- At the regional level, more than 11 million Africans have already died, and another 22 million are now living with HIV/AIDS. That is two-thirds of all the cases presently on earth.
- At the national level, the 21 countries with the highest HIV prevalence are in Africa. In Botswana and Zimbabwe, one in four adults is infected. In at least 10 other African countries, prevalence rates among adults exceed 10 percent.
- At the individual level, the arithmetic of risk is horrific. A child born in Zambia or Zimbabwe today is more likely than not to die of AIDS. In many other African countries, the lifetime risk of dying of AIDS is greater than one in three.

In short, as a result of the HIV/AIDS epidemic, much of Africa will enter the 21st century watching the gains of the 20th evaporate.

Tragically, mass killers are nothing new in Africa. Malaria still claims about as many African lives as AIDS, and preventable childhood diseases kill millions of others. What sets AIDS apart, however, is its unprecedented impact on regional development. Because it kills so many adults in the prime of their working and parenting lives, it decimates the workforce, fractures and impoverishes families, orphans millions, and shreds the fabric of communities. The costs it imposes force countries to make heartbreaking choices between today's and future lives, and between health and dozens of other vital investments for development. Given these realities, African governments and their partners must act now to prevent further HIV infections and to care for and support the millions of Africans already infected and affected.

The World Bank can and will play a stronger role in this effort. This document, *Intensifying Action Against HIV/AIDS in Africa: Responding to a Development Crisis,* introduces the Bank's new strategy to combat the epidemic in partnership with African governments and the Joint United Nations Programme on HIV/AIDS (UNAIDS). The strategy, approved by the Regional Leadership Team in May 1999, stands on four pillars:

- Advocacy to position HIV/AIDS as a central development issue and to increase and sustain an intensified response.
- Increased resources and technical support for African partners and Bank country teams to mainstream HIV/AIDS activities in all sectors.
- Prevention efforts targeted to both general and specific audiences, and activities to enhance HIV/AIDS treatment and care.
- Expanded knowledge base to help countries design and manage prevention, care, and treatment programs based on epidemic trends, impact forecasts, and identified best practices.

(An ideal national program that incorporates these four pillars is presented as a case study in Annex 1.)

To stimulate and support implementation of the strategy, the Bank has established a multisectoral AIDS Campaign Team for Africa (ACT*africa*), which will be based in the Office of the Regional Vice Presidents. The high-level placement of ACT*africa* underscores the Bank's commitment to HIV/AIDS prevention and care and will enable the team to maximize collaboration among the sector families. Most of ACT*africa*'s work will be demand-driven and funded from country budgets. The team will serve as the region's focal point and clearinghouse on HIV/AIDS and will provide a variety of services, including:

- Equipping and supporting Bank country teams to mobilize African leaders, civil society, and the private sector to intensify action against HIV/AIDS.
- Retrofitting projects with HIV/AIDS components where possible, assisting in the development of new dedicated HIV/AIDS projects, and building AIDS-mitigation measures into other projects where necessary.
- Supporting Bank country teams in addressing HIV/AIDS in their country assistance strategies.

- Exploring the feasibility of building an AIDS impact assessment module into existing environmental and/or social assessment processes.
- Collecting and disseminating information on the progress of the epidemics, country-by-country statistics, and best practices.
- Strengthening and expanding the Bank's partnership with UNAIDS, as well as with key agencies, nongovernmental organizations, and interested bilaterals.

The strategic plan detailed herein represents the Bank's next important step in the fight against HIV/AIDS in Africa. By its terms, we will now place HIV/AIDS at the center of our development agenda, and mainstream it in all aspects of our work in Africa and in all channels of our dialogue. We will help our clients intensify and expand their national responses and help build capacity among our staff in all sectors to factor HIV/AIDS into policies and projects. We will establish HIV/AIDS as both a corporate priority and our primary partnership issue. Finally, we will ensure that Sub-Saharan Africa realizes the full potential of our strategic partnership with UNAIDS.

It is easy to despair of AIDS. But let us bear in mind the many formidable challenges that Africa has already faced and overcome: wars of independence, global economic upheaval, droughts, floods. Then let us remember that unlike any of these, *AIDS is completely preventable.*

Recently, a history of the World Bank's first 50 years was published. In its more than 1,900 pages, including a 100-page chapter on Africa, the word "AIDS" barely appears. A generation from now, when the next such history is written, we can be certain that the pandemic will play a far more prominent role. Those who look back on this era will judge our institution in large measure by whether we recognized this wildfire that is raging across Africa for the development threat that it is, and did our utmost to put it out. They will be right to do so.

Let's get to work.

CALLISTO MADAVO
JEAN-LOUIS SARBIB

VICE PRESIDENTS
AFRICA REGION

JUNE 1999

Acknowledgments

This strategic plan was prepared by a team led by Debrework Zewdie (Lead Specialist, Africa Region and HIV/AIDS Coordinator, World Bank), comprising Sheila Mitchell and Sheila Dutta. Birger Fredriksen (Director, Human Development, Africa Region) and Ruth Kagia (Sector Manager, Human Development I, Africa Region) provided overall guidance.

The personal commitment of the Regional Vice Presidents, Callisto Madavo and Jean-Louis Sarbib, enabled the Regional Leadership Team to place HIV/AIDS at the center of the strategic agenda for Africa.

This document benefited from the invaluable guidance provided by the Intensifying Action Against HIV/AIDS Steering Committee: Hans Binswanger, Robert Calderisi, Abdou Salaam Drabo, Jacob Gayle, Salim Habayeb, Demissie Habte, Keith Hansen, Ohene Owusu Nyanin, A. Mead Over, Ok Pannenborg, and Albertus Voetberg. Of this group, Hans Binswanger, Robert Calderisi, Keith Hansen, and Albertus Voetberg drafted sections of the document. A review committee consisting of Pamela Cox, Alan Gelb, Letitia Obeng, and Hasan Tuluy provided valuable comments.

We also thank the many other Bank staff, the UNAIDS Secretariat and Cosponsoring Agencies, and the HNP External Advisory Panel for sharing their insights. The assistance of the UNAIDS Secretariat in providing us with data and the included maps is gratefully acknowledged.

We also would like to thank Robert Ritzenthaler for his assistance in editing this document.

A grant from the Norwegian Royal Ministry of Foreign Affairs enabled the preparation of this strategic plan.

Acronyms and Abbreviations

ACTafrica	AIDS Campaign Team for Africa
AIDS	acquired immunodeficiency syndrome
ARV	antiretroviral therapy
CAS	country assistance strategy
CBO	community-based organization
CILSS	Comité Inter-Etats de Lutte Contre la Séchéresse dans le Sahel
ESW	economic and sector work
HIPC	heavily indebted poor countries
HIV	human immunodeficiency virus
IAVI	International AIDS Vaccine Initiative
IBRD	International Bank for Reconstruction and Development
IDA	International Development Association
MTCT	mother-to-child transmission
NGO	nongovernmental organization
OAU	Organization for African Unity
OD	operational directive
OP	operational policy
SADC	Southern Africa Development Community
SSA	Sub-Saharan Africa
STI	sexually transmitted infection
UNAIDS	Joint United Nations Programme on HIV/AIDS
UNICEF	United Nations Children's Fund
UNDP	United Nations Development Programme
UNESCO	United Nations Education, Scientific, and Cultural Organization
UNFPA	United Nations Population Fund
VCT	voluntary counseling and testing
WHO	World Health Organization

1
Executive Summary

Two-thirds of the world's HIV/AIDS epidemic is in Africa. Last year alone, the disease killed 1.5 million people. They were not statistics. They were fathers and mothers, brothers and sisters, doctors and nurses, primary school teachers, electrical engineers, community leaders, finance managers, entrepreneurs, students, researchers, and farmers trying to lift their families out of poverty. Their spouses and children are now condemned to new hardship.

These people died because of the unique concentration of HIV in Africa, but also because the continent's leaders—and its international partners—have been slow to respond to the epidemic. Not since the bubonic plague of the European Middle Ages has there been so large a threat to hundreds of millions of people—and to the future of entire economies and societies.

Given the scale of the epidemic, it is no longer just a public health problem. It is a development crisis. And it has been in the making for at least 10 years. But challenges on so many fronts, the lack of knowledge about what to do, and a certain fatalism have overtaken the valiant efforts of a large number of people in Africa to make a dent in the massive infection rates. These people need fresh hope and new resources. Now is the time to act—and to act decisively.

This strategic plan calls on the World Bank, its development partners, and African governments to make a new commitment to saving millions of people from the worst effects of HIV/AIDS. This commitment will need to be as broad as the epidemic itself and intense enough to make up for a late start.

In particular, it calls on African leaders, civil society, and the private sector to put the HIV/AIDS crisis at the center of their national agendas. The Bank can raise the issue in international forums, conduct assessments on the impact of HIV/AIDS on development, sponsor international and regional conferences, and identify credible business leaders who can promote AIDS prevention in the workplace. The Bank can also help by identifying African elders and former statesmen, writers, musicians, artists, and athletes who would be willing to visit the worst-affected countries and dramatize the need for early action—particularly among young people.

The plan calls for building capacity within national and local governments, communities, and the private sector to design and implement effective programs. The Bank can help by providing technical assistance to countries; expanding existing management training programs to include national staff dealing with HIV/AIDS; and modifying existing Bank-financed projects (or developing new ones) to build capacity for HIV/AIDS prevention and care.

The Bank will need to strengthen its own capacity to respond to country requests for support by making HIV/AIDS a central element of its development agenda for Africa; providing timetables and guidance for Bank country teams to address the subject in all their projects and activities; including HIV/AIDS as an aspect of all country assistance strategies (CASs); requiring AIDS impact assessments for all projects; and issuing a Bank operational directive (OD) on the subject.

The Bank must also give its own staff the knowledge, tools, and resources needed to mobilize others by establishing an AIDS Campaign Team, ACTafrica, to provide operational support in all sectors; expanding such support into Bank country offices; developing analytical tools and briefs for Bank country teams to use with their country counterparts; collecting and disseminating information on intervention options and success stories; providing adequate resources to Bank country teams; and maintaining up-to-date Web pages on best practices.

Equally important will be continued Bank efforts to help countries improve their economic and social circumstances and hence slow the spread of the epidemic by educating girls; reducing poverty; making health sector reform more HIV/AIDS-sensitive; expanding gender initiatives; and strengthening capacity building to address the massive loss of skills and experience that has resulted from the epidemic.

The Bank should expand the resources available for fighting HIV/AIDS through increased funding for prevention, care, and treatment; redirecting ongoing project funds; using innovative mechanisms (such as social funds) for delivering resources to local governments, communities, and nongovernmental organizations (NGOs); and including HIV/AIDS among activities financed from the Heavily Indebted Poor Countries (HIPC) Trust Fund.

Bank-financed projects can also be retrofitted to reach more vulnerable populations and address long-term needs created by HIV/AIDS by supporting social assessment and impact studies to develop long-range planning; integrating information about HIV/AIDS into existing school and training curricula; and including condom distribution, treatment of sexually transmitted infections (STIs), and care and support into existing projects employing workers vulnerable to the disease.

The Bank must also mobilize additional resources from the international community through high-level meetings; better collaboration with the Joint United Nations Programme on HIV/AIDS (UNAIDS), other United Nations agencies, and international donors; and greater engagement with the international private sector.

Finally, the Bank should identify new ways of financing the development of affordable vaccines and other prevention options, such as microbicides, and support research efforts to provide decisionmakers with the data and tools they need to intensify their efforts against the epidemic.

HIV/AIDS has already reversed 30 years of hard-won social progress in some countries. Now is the time for Africa—and the world—to fight back.

2
The Gathering Storm

The Rapidly Growing HIV/AIDS Epidemic

The spread of HIV/AIDS has exceeded the worst projections by far. Nearly 34 million people in the world are currently living with HIV/AIDS, and one-third of these are young people between the ages of 10 and 24. The epidemic continues to grow, as 16,000 people worldwide become newly infected each day. Fourteen million adults and children have already lost their lives to this devastating disease, and the death toll rises each year (UNAIDS, 1998e). Despite these alarming figures, AIDS is still an emerging and growing epidemic.

The region most affected has been Sub-Saharan Africa (SSA). (In this document, "Africa" and "Sub-Saharan Africa" are used interchangeably.) At the end of 1998, 22.5 million people, including 1 million children, were living with HIV/AIDS in SSA, two-thirds of the worldwide total (Figure 1). At least 4 million Africans were newly infected with the virus in 1998. HIV does not respect borders, and its transmission is often facilitated by subregional trade routes and other migration patterns common throughout the continent. In Botswana, Namibia, Zambia, and Zimbabwe, between 20 and 26 percent of people ages 15 to 49 are infected. In 12 other SSA countries, including Ethiopia, Kenya, Mozambique, South Africa, and Tanzania, 9 to 20 percent of adults are infected (UNAIDS, 1998a; Annex 2). Some countries in West and Central Africa have been less affected and have been able to maintain low and stable HIV infection rates. This is due, in part, to an early response to the threat of the epidemic in some countries, and in part because a less virulent HIV strain (HIV-2) predominates in these countries. However, there is no single factor or clear-cut group of factors that determines the severity of a country's HIV/AIDS epidemic.

Deaths due to HIV/AIDS in Africa will soon surpass the 20 million Europeans killed by the plague epidemic of 1347–1351 (Decosas and Adrien, 1999).

It is estimated that only 10 percent of the illness and death that this epidemic will bring has been seen. The real impact on people, communities, and economies is still to come. There is no affordable cure or vaccine likely to be available in developing countries for a decade or more. The only

Figure 1. *Global and Sub-Saharan Africa Disease Burden, December 1998 (Millions)*

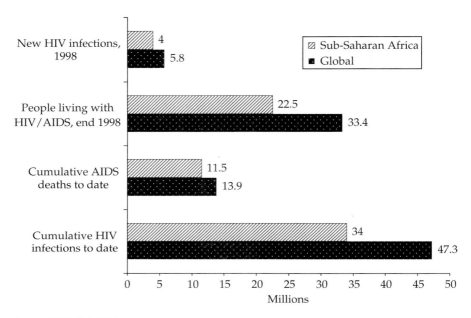

Source: UNAIDS, 1998e.

options are to prevent further spread of the epidemic, minimize its impact, and provide a caring and compassionate environment for those infected and affected. This crisis calls for an expanded and intensified response to mobilize governments, civil society, the private sector, and the international community to take action, increase resources, and build capacity to sustain efforts to slow the spread of the epidemic.

HIV/AIDS' Devastating Impact on Development

The HIV/AIDS epidemic is not only the most important public health problem affecting large parts of SSA, but also an unprecedented threat to the region's development. It is, therefore, a development crisis.

The most disturbing long-term feature of the HIV/AIDS epidemic is its impact on life expectancy, making HIV an unprecedented catastrophe in the world's history. Among 18 countries in SSA that experienced a declining or stagnating life expectancy during 1990–1995, all but one (Togo) were described as having a generalized HIV/AIDS epidemic, that is, an HIV prevalence of more than 5 percent in the adult population. Conversely, of 29 countries that experienced an improvement in life expectancy, only two, Mozambique and Lesotho, had a generalized epidemic (World Bank, 1999).

In nine African countries with adult prevalence of 10 percent or more, HIV/AIDS will erase 17 years of potential gains in life expectancy, meaning that instead of reaching 64 years, by 2010–2015 life expectancy in these countries will regress to an average of just 47 years; this represents a reversal of most development gains of the past 30 years—affecting an entire generation (UNAIDS, 1998e). Figure 2 indicates estimated life expectancy in selected African countries.

HIV/AIDS is also surpassing malaria as the leading cause of death in many countries (Figure 3).

Demographic projections vary in predicting the effects of the epidemic on population growth. However, all agree that there will be a decrease in annual population growth in the region by 2010. It is unlikely that the epidemic in any country will reach proportions severe enough and cause a rapid enough decline in fertility to exhibit a negative population growth due to HIV (Decosas and Adrien, 1999).

Figure 2. *Estimated Life Expectancy at Birth: Selected African Countries, 1955–2000*

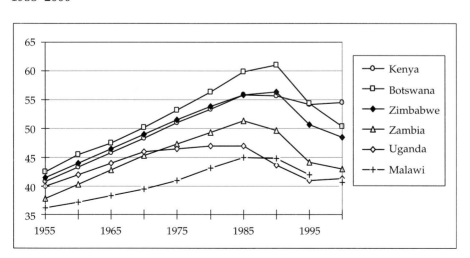

Source: UNAIDS, 1998a.

Figure 3. *Adult Deaths from Infectious Diseases in the Developing World, 1990 and 2020.*

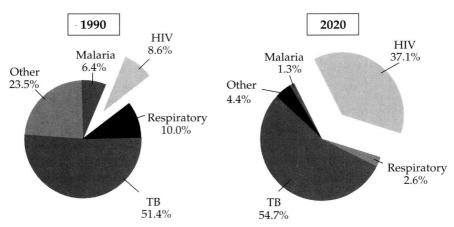

Source: World Bank, 1997a.

Child mortality is rising. In 1998, about 530,000 HIV-infected children were born in SSA, about 90 percent of the world total. By 2005–2010, infant mortality in South Africa will be 60 percent higher than it would have been without HIV/AIDS (61 deaths per 1,000 infants born rather than 38 per 1,000 in the absence of AIDS). In Zambia and Zimbabwe, 25 percent more infants are already dying than would be the case without HIV. By 2010, Zimbabwe's infant and child mortality rates will have doubled (UNAIDS, 1998e).

Young people are disproportionately affected. Worldwide, about half of all new HIV infections occur in young people ages 15 to 24. In 1998, nearly 3 million young people became infected with the virus, equivalent to more than five young men and women every minute of the day, every day of the year (UNAIDS, 1998a). Girls become infected younger and die earlier than boys due to age asymmetry in sexual partnerships. In countries such as Ethiopia, Malawi, Tanzania, Zambia, and Zimbabwe, for every 15- to 19-year-old boy who is infected, there are five to six girls infected in the same age group.

The disease mainly strikes people in their prime years. Worldwide, AIDS hits people hardest in their most productive years. This profoundly disrupts the economic and social bases of families. When a family loses its primary income earner, its very survival is threatened. It sells assets and exhausts savings to pay for health care and funerals.

Children are being orphaned in huge numbers. In 1997, approximately 1.5 million children in SSA were orphaned by the disease. (UNAIDS has defined orphans as children under 15 who have lost their mother or both parents to AIDS.) To date, there are 7.8 million AIDS orphans in this region alone. In some hard-hit cities, orphans comprise 15 percent of all children (UNAIDS, 1998a). Care for these orphans often falls on extended families, stretching the capacity of these social safety nets. Many orphans are now heading households. They are far less likely to attend school, more likely to be undernourished, less likely to receive immunizations or health care, and usually very poor. Orphans often end up on the streets, where they pursue survival strategies that put them at great risk of contracting HIV themselves (USAID, 1997).

National income is affected. The illness and impending death of up to 25 percent of all adults in some countries will have an enormous impact on national productivity and earnings. Labor productivity is likely to drop, the benefits of education will be lost, and resources that would have been used for investments will be used for health care, orphan care, and funerals. Savings rates will decline, and the loss of human capital will affect production and the quality of life for years to come. Countries need to plan for the human resource needs that will result from the millions of premature deaths.

The epidemic is having a tremendous subregional impact. Southern Africa has one of the world's most rapidly spreading HIV/AIDS epidemics. The eight countries with the highest prevalence rates in the world (see Annex 2), ranging from 12 to 25 percent of the adult population, are in Southern Africa. Zimbabwe is especially hard hit with up to 50 percent of pregnant women in some sites infected. In Botswana, Namibia, and Zambia, the prevalence rates among pregnant women are between 20 and 40 percent. South Africa trailed behind many of its neighbors in 1990 but is rapidly catching up. In 1998, South Africa accounted for over half of all new infections in Southern Africa and for one in seven new infections in SSA. The socioeconomic costs of South Africa's HIV/AIDS epidemic are critical not just within the country itself, but for its neighbors as well, given the interconnectedness of many economies to the economy of South Africa and the high degree of movement among countries in the subregion.

Impact of the Epidemic on Various Sectors

Many studies have tried to demonstrate the macroeconomic impact of the HIV/AIDS epidemic, but the interaction between the epidemic and economic performance is complex (Decosas and Adrien, 1999). Other studies have been able to provide a more detailed view of the economic consequences of the epidemic in the industry and economic sectors, geographic regions, and specific demographic groups.

Social safety nets and impact on households. The HIV/AIDS epidemic is stretching the capacity of social safety nets to the limit. The numbers of AIDS patients, widows, and orphans are growing rapidly. The household impacts begin as soon as a member of the household starts to suffer from HIV-related illness. This results in loss of income of the patient, a substantial increase in household expenditures for medical expenses, and other members of the household, usually daughters and wives, missing school or work to care for the sick person. Death results not only in additional expenses for funeral and mourning costs, but also in a permanent loss of income from less labor on the farm or from lower remittances. Poor households are more vulnerable to the impact of an AIDS death, which significantly affects food expenditure and consumption and ultimately impacts childhood nutrition (World Bank, 1997a). Death of a parent often results in removal of children from school to save educational expenses and increase household labor, resulting in a severe loss of future earning potential. Widows in particular may have no means to support themselves after their husbands die, which often forces them into commercial sex work and increases their risk of infection. The large number of orphans in Africa is not only a major development problem; the increasing number of children-headed households   is creating a new social system with inherent problems that societies have yet to address. This growing crisis is putting pressure on governments to increasingly support safety nets where they exist or create effective social safety nets where they do not. Greater investment in social programs and strengthening of institutions to deal with these growing needs will help construct these social safety nets.

Health care. Maintaining a healthy population is an important goal in its own right and is crucial to the development of a productive workforce, which, in turn, is essential for economic development. The countries most affected by AIDS are often those least able to afford increased costs of health care. Health care systems are stretched beyond their limits as they not only deal with a growing number of AIDS patients and the loss of health personnel due to death and illness, but also cope with rising cases of tuberculosis, the most common opportunistic infection associated with AIDS. Tuberculosis adds to the burden of illness and shortens life expectancy (UNAIDS, 1997b). In Côte d'Ivoire, Zambia, and Zimbabwe, HIV-infected patients occupy 50 to 80 percent of all beds in urban hospitals. The services provided meet only a fraction of the needs. Yet spending on AIDS care is crowding out spending on other lifesaving, cost-effective programs. On average, treating an AIDS patient for one year is about as expensive as educating 10 primary school students for one year (World Bank, 1997a). There is little hope that any development goals for health (such as reduced infant, child, and maternal mortality, or reduced mortality from malaria) can be achieved in the face of AIDS. The motivation and incentive system for health workers needs to be reviewed from the perspectives of both service delivery and overall sectoral objectives. AIDS also poses significant challenges for health sector reform and is dramatically changing the disease burden profile in many countries (UNAIDS, 1998c). It is bound to change the components of essential health care packages as well. Effective strategies are needed to find and strengthen alternatives to hospital care for patients suffering from AIDS as well as to assist in procuring much-needed drugs and supplies for treatment.

Education. AIDS is reducing the hard-won returns on investment in education and exacting a staggering human cost. Scarce resources spent on education will be lost if teachers and students die of AIDS—the more skilled, the greater the economic loss. Millions of teachers and students are dying or leaving school for economic reasons, because of illness, or to care for family members, reducing both the demand for education and the supply of teachers. More than 30 percent of teachers in Malawi and Zambia are already infected (UNAIDS, 1998b). Infected parents keep children (especially girls) out of school for economic and social reasons, presenting an increasing challenge to reach these out-of-school youth with effective AIDS-prevention programs. That young girls are particularly at risk of contracting HIV, undermines their hopes for education. The resulting lower female education will undermine recent gains in health, nutrition, and family planning. AIDS also affects education at higher levels. Firms grow reluctant to invest in training as the turnover among workers rapidly rises. The education sector has a key role in promoting and maintaining the critical behavior-change agenda and must take these factors into account when planning. Educators must seek every opportunity to include HIV/AIDS prevention in school and training curricula at all levels.

Agriculture. Agriculture is the largest sector in most African economies, accounting for a large portion of production and employing the majority of workers. Many of the countries most affected by HIV/AIDS are heavily reliant on agriculture and agricultural exports to pay for raw materials and essential imports for development. Coping strategies developed by rural communities affected by HIV can lead to greater poverty and increased vulnerability. The loss of adults to AIDS often leads to a shift in cropping patterns. In many cases, this means switching from cash crops to subsistence farming. It can also reduce investments in soil enhancements, irrigation, and other capital improvements, which have long-term impacts on output. AIDS forces families to make irreversible decisions to sell livestock, equipment, and land to cover AIDS-related expenses, leaving surviving family members in poverty, from which it is hard to escape (Topouzis, 1998). In addition, agricultural knowledge and management skills are being lost. A study conducted with the Zimbabwe Farmers Union showed that the death of a breadwinner due to AIDS will cut the production of maize in small-scale farming and communal areas by 61 percent (The Policy Project, 1999). In Malawi, where 10 percent of gross domestic product comes from estate agriculture, the strongest effect of HIV/AIDS will be the negative impact on the supply of skilled labor (The Policy Project, 1999). Bank country teams must examine the long-term impact of AIDS as it spreads to rural areas and address these issues now in long-term planning and resource development. Proven HIV/AIDS-prevention tools can be incorporated into agriculture training programs and extended through existing mechanisms such as extension agents to reach the many rural people who are vulnerable to the epidemic.

Infrastructure and mining. Mining and construction of roads, dams, bridges, and other infrastructure often take workers away from their families. This increases the risk of HIV infection for both workers and people living near the construction sites. A study in Ghana has found prevalence of HIV infection to be 5 to 10 percent higher in a rural district where the Akosomo hydroelectric dam was under construction than in neighboring districts. Not only did construction of the dam draw workers away from their families and increase commercial sex work in the area, but it also displaced 80,000 inhabitants (Decosas, 1996). The potential for infrastructure projects to contribute to the spread of AIDS needs to be considered in project design, whereby these projects are used as an opportunity to extend HIV-prevention efforts. AIDS prevention and care for workers, their families, and the surrounding communities must be incorporated into all infrastructure and mining projects to reduce potential impact and expand prevention coverage. The World Bank and others can play an important role in enlisting the private sector to accept this responsibility.

Private sector firms. AIDS-related illnesses and deaths to employees affect private sector firms by increasing expenditures and reducing revenues. Industries that rely on a high level of skilled labor and are in an environment of high HIV prevalence are most vulnerable. The main effect of HIV on industry is through increased labor costs and decreased availability of skilled labor (Decosas and Adrien, 1999). Numerous countries in Africa are facing the prospect of significant increases in staff costs arising from absenteeism (due to illness and family bereavements), higher labor turnover (due to illness and deaths), and increasing recruitment, training, and staff welfare costs (medical insurance, medical expenses, and benefits to employees).

A study examining several firms in Botswana and Kenya demonstrated
that the most significant factors in increased labor costs were absenteeism
due to HIV/AIDS and increased burial costs (Roberts and Rau, 1997).
HIV/AIDS is costing Kenyan companies an average of US$25 per employee annually. These costs, which result from absenteeism and increased
expenditures for medical and other benefits, are expected to increase to an
average of US$56 by 2005 if the rate of HIV incidence continues unchecked.
Conversely, a comprehensive prevention program in Kenya would cost an
estimated US$15 per employee annually (UNAIDS, 1998e). It is critical to
convince the private sector to join the national response to the epidemic and
address these issues in their planning, as well as take responsibility for prevention and care of their workers.

The Imperative of Urgent Action

The cost of inaction. Although prevention strategies were known early in the
course of the epidemic and many interventions have been implemented on
a limited scale, only a few countries have taken sufficient action to curtail the
spread of HIV/AIDS. Inaction to date has resulted in millions of new infections and unnecessary deaths, leading to the current crisis situation that will
require considerable effort and resources to bring the epidemic under control.

In 1982, there was only one country in Africa, Uganda, with an adult HIV
prevalence rate higher than 2 percent. Today there are 21 countries in Africa
with prevalence rates of more than 7 percent. Since 1985, the prevalence of
HIV in urban antenatal women in Blantyre, Malawi, has increased from less
than 5 percent to over 30 percent. In Francistown, Botswana, reported rates
in antenatal women were less than 10 percent as recently as 1991 but rose to
43 percent in 1997 (U.S. Bureau of the Census, 1998). In Ethiopia, the proportion of adults infected with HIV increased from less than 1 percent to
nearly 10 percent between 1987 and 1997. These alarming figures illustrate
how quickly the epidemic can spread out of control.

The cost of delaying an intensified response is monumental. More than 4
million people in SSA were newly infected in 1998, and the numbers are certain to grow in 1999. Most of these people will die within the next decade,
leaving millions of orphans. The resulting social decay and breakdown will
threaten socioeconomic development for decades to come.

The benefit of action. Despite the mounting crisis, the situation is far from
hopeless. Although HIV prevalence rates are high, more than 200 million
adults in Africa are not yet infected. However, many are vulnerable and

will be infected and die unless action is taken now.

Studies have shown that specific interventions using voluntary counseling and testing (VCT), condom social marketing, peer education, and treatment of sexually transmitted infections (STIs) can change behaviors and reduce the risk of HIV. Modeling has shown that the synergistic effect of combining these interventions reduces the risks even further. The following pilot projects were carefully evaluated and demonstrate the effect these specific interventions can have on changing behavior and reducing transmission of STIs, including HIV:

- Results of a Rwandan study on the impact of preventive counseling and testing indicated that for women whose partners were also tested and counseled, the annual incidence of new HIV infections decreased from 4.1 percent to 1.8 percent. Among women who were HIV-positive, the prevalence of gonorrhea decreased from 13 percent to 6 percent, with the greatest reduction in those using condoms (Allen and others, 1992). The estimated cost of VCT programs in SSA is US$4.40 per person counseled and tested. (The cost estimates provided in these examples are not specific to these studies but were compiled from the literature on costs of interventions througout SSA and represent a medium-cost scenario; Kmaranayake and Watts, 1999).

- An intervention in the Democratic Republic of Congo targeted education, STI treatment, and condoms to commercial sex workers, resulting in an increase in regular condom use with clients from 10 to 68 percent in three years. The incidence of HIV dropped from 11.7 to 4.4 per 100 person-years of observation, and there was a decline in the incidence of treatable STIs (Laga and others, 1994). The estimated cost of STI treatment is approximately US$2.33 per case.

- A condom social marketing program in Brazil resulted in a reduction in the price of condoms from US$.075 to US$.020. Under this program, the total market volume for condoms more than tripled from 45 million to 168 million in four years (World Bank, 1997a). It is estimated that each condom distributed through a social marketing program in SSA costs approximately US$0.25 to US$0.34.

- A project in Kenya distributed condoms and educational materials and provided STI treatment to male truck drivers through a workplace intervention. After one year, there was a reported 13 percent decrease in extramarital sex (49 percent to 36 percent) and a 6 percent decrease in visits to commercial sex workers (12 percent to 6 percent). There was also a decline in STIs (Jackson and others, 1997). Other studies have estimated the cost of a workplace intervention focusing only on education to be US$0.50 per worker reached. The costs of STI treatment and condoms would be similar to those noted above.

- Studies in Mwanza, Tanzania, show that early, continuous treatment of STIs in a rural community was associated with a 42 percent decline in newly acquired HIV infections at a cost of US$10 per person treated (Grosskurth and others, 1995). More recent evidence indicates that STI control may be most effective in the early phase of an HIV epidemic (Wawer and others, 1999).

The challenge is to incorporate these and other effective interventions into a comprehensive national program, bring them to scale, and sustain them. By so doing, certain countries have been able to slow the epidemic and minimize its impact. These countries have been able to change social norms to help people lower their risk of HIV and have significantly reduced the number of new infections. The active response and success of HIV-prevention efforts in these countries provide reason for hope:

- There were significant decreases in HIV prevalence among women attending prenatal clinics in certain regions of Uganda between 1990–1993 and 1994–1995. These were noted particularly among women ages 15 to 24 (Wawer and others, 1999). Strong, high-level, national leadership and effective partnerships with civil society facilitated the changes leading to this decrease.
- The leadership of Senegal chose not to deny the existence of the epidemic, but to face the challenge from the start. Enlisting all key actors as allies in a timely and aggressive prevention campaign has helped the country maintain one of the lowest HIV-infection rates in SSA (1.77 percent). The small number of HIV-positive individuals allows the government to consider utilizing treatment schedules that otherwise would not have been affordable (UNAIDS, 1998e).
- Numerous Western countries have established and sustained comprehensive HIV/AIDS-prevention efforts that have greatly reduced the spread of the epidemic. The most notable features of the Australian response to HIV/AIDS are support from all political parties and strong partnerships among community groups, government officials, health workers, the private sector, and researchers (National Centre in HIV Epidemiology and Clinical Research, 1997). The Swiss strategy highlights the vitality of developing strong working partnerships with people living with HIV/AIDS, local and regional officials, and nongovernmental organizations (Swiss Federal Office of

Public Health, 1999). The response to HIV/AIDS in the Netherlands has been comprehensive and progressive, particularly with respect to its community-based outreach programs and partnerships with groups at increased risk of HIV infection.

- In Thailand, concerted government prevention efforts at the national and regional levels led to a rapid and sharp decline in new HIV and sexually transmitted infections. As can be seen in Figure 4, the number of male STI cases decreased dramatically as condom use among sex workers rose.

Figure 4. *The Impact of Rising Condom Use in Thailand*

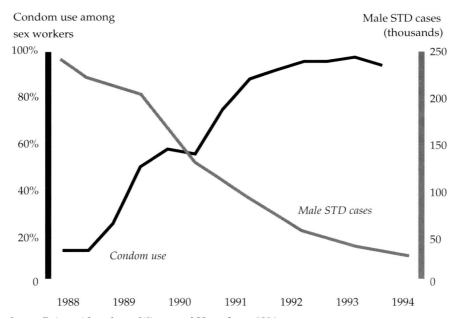

Source: Rojanapithayakorn, Wiwat, and Hanenberg, 1996.

3
Building an
Effective Response

Governments must rally and invest early in the epidemic, recognizing the unique epidemic characteristics in each country and the determinants of epidemic spread. Prevention is much less expensive than treatment and avoids the sickness, death, and socioeconomic impact that will ultimately result (World Bank, 1997a). Although AIDS has already resulted in severe deterioration in the economic and social conditions of many SSA countries, there is much that can be done now to halt the epidemic and mitigate its impact. Necessary responses include the following.

Intensify, Expand, and Improve the National Response

An expanded, multisectoral, and national response will extend the reach of current prevention efforts to those who are vulnerable and will reduce the impact of the epidemic on all sectors. It will address the biological, behavioral, and social factors that determine the profile of the epidemic in each country. The key components of effective HIV-prevention programs include changing individual behavior and social norms to reduce risk, making condoms available and affordable, providing effective diagnosis and treatment of STIs, ensuring a safe blood supply, and supporting affordable interventions to reduce transmission from mother to child. Focusing comprehensive efforts on the groups most at risk of contracting and spreading HIV has been necessary and cost-effective in all successful efforts. These components must be integrated into activities in all sectors. World Bank country teams must help countries understand the impact this epidemic will have on all sectors and adjust programs and project designs to take this fully into account.

Address the Root Causes of Vulnerability

Two major factors render a society vulnerable to a major HIV epidemic: (1) social destructuring as experienced during war, rapid economic or political changes, or massive migration; and (2) low social cohesion, which is a measure of a society's ability to cope with stress (Decosas and Adrien, 1999).

The HIV/AIDS epidemic disproportionately affects women, especially young girls, and the poor. The impact of AIDS on households can be reduced to some extent by putting programs in place to address specific problems. For example:

- Improved economic opportunities, gender-sensitive legal and regulatory frameworks, and elimination of harmful and discriminatory practices will improve the status of women and help them avoid infection.
- Educating children, especially girls, will enhance their ability to avoid infection.
- Reduced school fees can help children from poor families and AIDS orphans stay in school longer.
- Establishing outreach programs for street children and other out-of-school youth will help reduce HIV infection among this vulnerable group.
- Creative incentives for training can encourage firms to maintain worker productivity despite the loss of experienced workers.
- Home care for HIV/AIDS patients and support for basic needs of households can help families cope.
- Foster care for orphans, food programs for children, and support for educational expenses can help families and children survive some of the consequences of the epidemic.
- Social funds can help grassroots organizations cope.

Assess the Impact of Development Projects on HIV/AIDS

Major development projects may inadvertently facilitate the spread of HIV. For example, major construction projects often require large numbers of male workers to live apart from their families for extended periods of time, leading to increased opportunities for men to purchase commercial sex and to an increased likelihood that women left behind may resort to it for economic survival. These projects can be designed or retrofitted to reduce these risks by providing innovative means to keep families together, reduce mobility, generate income, and provide strong prevention programs.

Learn from Experience

Successful programs from Uganda to Australia and from Senegal to Thailand have shown that government commitment to creating an enabling environment for all partners is key. This is supported by a strong alliance with the private sector, communities, NGOs, and people infected and affected by HIV who have been leading the fight so far. Although much has been learned about how to curtail the epidemic, most countries are slow to act and have not been able to scale up successful interventions to reach all at-risk individuals. Governments must take the lead to scale up and intensify actions to a national level.

Worldwide, youth are disproportionately affected by this epidemic. This large and growing segment of the population also has been the most responsive to behavior-change interventions. Studies have shown that youth programs can make a significant and sustainable impact on this impressionable audience. A global assessment of school-based programs found that sexual health education and AIDS prevention incorporated into school-based programs not only delayed the start of sexual activity but also reduced the number of sexual partners and raised contraceptive use among those who became sexually active (UNAIDS, 1997a).

Public economics and epidemiologic principles argue strongly to intervene early and prevent infections among those most likely to catch and spread the virus to avert the largest number of new infections (World Bank, 1997a). The need to prioritize and effectively use scarce resources becomes even more important when a country brings successful interventions to national scale. To put effective programs in place, SSA countries have been divided into two major categories:[5]

1. *Countries with adult HIV prevalence rates of 7 percent or more.* Twenty-one (21) countries meet this criterion. In these countries, a strategy is required that continues to strengthen interventions targeted to groups at highest risk, and at the same time will lead to rapid coverage of all vulnerable groups in all urban areas and rural districts. These countries must also move rapidly beyond prevention to provide care and mitigate the impact of the epidemic.

2. *Countries with adult HIV prevalence rates of less than 7 percent.* Twenty-three (23) countries fall in this category. HIV in these countries remains predominantly in groups whose behavior places them at high risk, but it has the potential to spread rapidly to the general population. To contain the spread of the epidemic in these countries, priority should be given to changing the behavior of those at highest risk of contracting and spreading HIV. This sharply targeted effort needs to be national in scope and be quickly followed by broader approaches to reach other vulnerable groups, such as women and youth.

A strategy, national in scope, is therefore required in all countries. The strategy is initially more focused on prevention and on groups at highest risk in the low-prevalence countries. In the high-prevalence countries, the program must address wider objectives and reach all vulnerable groups while reinforcing sustainable behavior change among those at highest risk.

What works? Successful national HIV/AIDS programs have many things in common:

- They have government commitment at the highest level and multiple partnerships at all levels with civil society and the private sector.
- They invest early in effective prevention efforts.
- They require cooperation and collaboration among many different groups and sectors: those who are most affected by the epidemic, religious and community leaders, NGOs, researchers and health professionals, and the private sector.
- They are decentralized and use participatory approaches to bring prevention and care programs to truly national scale.
- The response is forward-looking, comprehensive, and multisectoral; addresses the socioeconomic determinants that make people vulnerable to infection; and targets prevention interventions and care and treatment support to them.
- They are characterized by community participation in government policymaking as well as design and implementation of programs; many of these are implemented by people living with HIV/AIDS, NGOs, civil society, and the private sector.

These national programs all focus on a core set of interventions that have been proven on a small scale to change behavior, to reduce the risk of HIV transmission, and to be cost-effective. These interventions can all be implemented through a strong partnership with the government, NGOs, civil society, people living with HIV/AIDS, and the private sector. They include:

- Changing behavior to reduce risks through communication, including mass media, peer education, theater, and counseling, especially among youth.
- Making STI diagnosis and treatment readily available and affordable.
- Treating opportunistic infections, including tuberculosis.
- Making condoms affordable and widely accessible.
- Ensuring a safe blood supply.
- Making voluntary counseling and testing (VCT) available and affordable.

- Preventing transmission from mother to child (see Annex 4).

An ideal program that incorporates these interventions is presented as a case study in Annex 1.

As the epidemic progresses, with over 22 million Africans already infected, the need to strengthen care, treatment, and social support becomes a high priority. Programs are needed to finance and implement home-, hospice-, and hospital-based care; treatment for opportunistic infections and STIs; and social support for those affected by AIDS, including widows and orphans. These strategies can help families, communities, and nations cope. Experience demonstrates that communities are often in the best position to launch a response to the epidemic and take care of their own. All they need are the enabling environment, the tools, and the resources.

What does not work? Many years of experience have shown that the following strategies do not work and that some can actually be damaging to program efforts:

- Expecting health-oriented national AIDS committees to lead an intensified response to the epidemic in the absence of adequate, sustained, and high-level government support.
- Undertaking centralized programs, led by ministries of health, primarily focusing on the health aspects of the epidemic.
- Inadequately targeting interventions to small sections of populations at increased risk of both HIV infection and transmission.
- Withholding knowledge from young people that would protect them from infection, under the guise of "cultural and social norms."
- Targeting the vulnerable, especially women and young girls, without addressing the root causes of their vulnerability.
- Stigmatizing and marginalizing those infected and affected by this epidemic.
- Investing in expensive pilot studies that have no chance of being sustained, replicated, or expanded.
- Building plans and programs that are externally driven, based on available funding or donor interest rather than well-coordinated programs based on need and proven strategies.
- Designing programs without community involvement.

Sporadic or isolated activities are ineffective unless they are evaluated as pilot activities and revised and expanded on the basis of what has been learned. To maximize their impact, programs should be implemented for long periods on the basis of need rather than funding cycles.

Focusing on information and education is not enough to reduce people's risk; it is essential to foster an environment that facilitates changes in social norms, address poverty, and provide the tools for people to change their behavior.

What does an ideal program look like and how much does it cost? A fully costed case study of an ideal national program is presented in Annex 1. The cost estimates are based on a costing model developed specifically for this strategy (Kumaranayake and Watts, 1999). Similar estimates have been developed for 24 countries in SSA and will soon be published under separate cover.

4

Strategic Plan
for Intensifying Action
against AIDS in Africa

This strategic plan builds upon the important partnerships of the World Bank with African countries, UNAIDS, the private sector, and donor agencies and summarizes the World Bank's contribution to the common framework for action agreed upon by UNAIDS. In this strategy, the Bank addresses the HIV/AIDS epidemic as a major development threat to SSA and defines the actions the Bank will take in support of the UNAIDS International Partnership Against HIV/AIDS in Africa (see Annex 3).

Goal

The goal of this strategic plan is to urgently assist African governments and mobilize the Bank, development partners, the private sector, and civil society to intensify action on multisectoral and sustainable policies and programs to address the compelling and evolving implications of the HIV/AIDS epidemic to halt further reversal of human, social, and economic development in Africa.

Approach

Together with UNAIDS, the Bank will intensify its actions against HIV/AIDS in Africa by providing the necessary resources and technical support to country teams to mainstream HIV/AIDS activities in all sectors. To reach the stated goal, the Bank's approach will stand on the following four pillars: advocacy; increased resources; programs for prevention, care, and treatment; and knowledge.

- Advocacy efforts targeted to policymakers at the national and international levels will increase and sustain the demand for an intensified action. These efforts will increase awareness within the Bank and

23

globally to position HIV/AIDS as a development issue and mobilize additional resources.

- Bank lending and economic and sector work (ESW) for HIV/AIDS have diminished to a trickle in recent years. This stems from the lack of progressive programs at the country level as well as from the narrowness of the Bank's present approaches to AIDS. To reverse this trend, the Bank needs to take a broader, more strategic, and more timely approach to integrating HIV/AIDS into existing activities. In collaboration with UNAIDS, the Bank will intensify its actions against AIDS in Africa by providing the necessary resources and technical support to Bank country teams to mainstream HIV/AIDS activities in all sectors.

- In countries with a more generalized epidemic (those with HIV prevalence rates of 7 percent or higher), the highest priority will be to increase the scale of prevention efforts to reach all people who are vulnerable and to rapidly build capabilities to provide care and treatment. In countries with relatively low prevalence rates (less than 7 percent), the highest priority will be to bring prevention efforts to a national scale, focusing on those whose behavior puts them at higher risk, and to identify and reinforce the social norms that seem to be preventing epidemic spread. To accomplish this, the Bank and its partners will provide Bank country teams with tools and financial resources to assess needs and provide support to their countries.

- There is a continuing need for information and data to increase the Bank's knowledge base. The response to this epidemic must evolve based on new information and solid data for decisionmaking. While expanding the global knowledge base is the responsibility of UNAIDS, this strategy will help expand the knowledge base of Bank staff to help countries design and manage prevention, care, and treatment programs based on epidemic trends, impact forecasts, and identified best practices. This information and data will also be used to inform leaders and motivate them to take action.

This strategy is a guiding document for the Bank's work in the Africa region. It is based on the comparative advantages of the Bank to lead efforts in advocacy, financing, and analysis in partnership with other development partners and in support of the UNAIDS International Partnership Against HIV/AIDS in Africa. This is a regional strategy involving multiple partners that provides the overarching framework for customizing involvement at the country level.

Overcoming Barriers

There is little disagreement about what works to slow the HIV/AIDS epidemic. The challenge is to create the enabling environment and mobilize the resources to quickly bring these interventions to scale. This strategy addresses the following constraints and provides the tools to overcome them:

- *Lack of strong political commitment.* Not all African leaders and development agencies are convinced of the seriousness of the epidemic, nor do they realize the potential impact it will have on their countries. Because of this, they have not made HIV/AIDS a high priority. A strong political commitment to the fight against AIDS is crucial to provide the needed resources, strong leadership, and enabling environment that are critical to controlling epidemic spread and caring for the nation. Accurate and relevant data are a powerful tool to convince leaders to increase their commitment to confronting this epidemic. These data are even more powerful when presented by respected international and regional peers. This strategy will primarily target countries that lack sufficient commitment and other key elements to mobilize them to take action.
- *Competing priorities.* Most countries in Africa must simultaneously address multiple serious health, political, economic, and social problems. Some leaders see HIV/AIDS as only an additional issue requiring more resources. Because the real impact of AIDS is not felt immediately, leaders find it difficult to respond at an early stage of the epidemic when preventive measures are most effective. Appropriate use of relevant data and modeling techniques is critical to helping leaders visualize the impact the epidemic will have on all sectors and to placing it within the context of the competing priorities.
- *Insufficient resources and inadequate capacity to mount the necessary level of response.* Although the epidemic is generalized in most African countries and reaching well beyond those groups with high-risk behaviors, most current programs are not reaching nearly enough people in rural areas, especially youth and women. Few countries have sufficient human and financial resources to mount a full-scale program. Governments must work with their partners to leverage additional funding and continually build and replenish capacity within their countries to sustain an expanded response. Governments must also give support to NGOs, community groups, and people living with HIV/AIDS to expand their capacity.

- *"Cultural norms" or religious beliefs.* Some countries are reluctant to acknowledge that certain practices, such as commercial sex work and intravenous drug use, exist in their country and will not address the serious risks that these practices pose. Some are reluctant to change behaviors that are part of the "cultural norms," such as female genital mutilation, even when these behaviors place people at risk of HIV infection. And yet others will not address sensitive issues such as sexual health of adolescents because of strong traditions and irrational fears. The approach to mobilizing leaders in these countries is to customize the strategies, bringing religious and traditional leaders on board, to gradually address the obstacles and build a positive response. Countries can learn from others with similar cultural or religious constraints and conduct operations research and pilot studies to evaluate new approaches.

Actions

The following actions describe the substance of what the Bank will do in collaboration with its partners to fight the HIV/AIDS epidemic during the next five years. A detailed implementation plan will be developed within the next six months that will describe how to bring these actions to scale and present various financing options. Detailed descriptions of activities at the international, regional, and country levels are presented below.

The Bank and its partners will be able to initiate these actions only if countries in SSA are willing to lead the intensified action and request assistance. Only then will this strategy effectively be supporting sustainable programs owned by the countries themselves.

1.   Increase Demand to Intensify Action

1.a.   Assist African Leaders to Mobilize Civil Society and the Private Sector to Intensify Action against AIDS within Their Countries

The leadership for intensified action against HIV/AIDS must come from the countries themselves. The governments of these countries should foster a strong alliance with civil society and the private sector to ensure that the response is truly effective and sustainable. The Bank can assist in mobilizing African nations to intensify their action against HIV/AIDS through a variety of measures.

- *Identify influential leaders to mobilize others.* The Bank has access to the highest-level decisionmakers in SSA and should use this access to persuade leaders to take action. Apart from the Bank's president, regional vice presidents, and executive directors, it can organize teams composed of African elders, former statesmen, opinion leaders, and friends of Africa that will visit countries that request assistance and demonstrate readiness to intensify their response to HIV/AIDS. The teams will meet with high-level government officials, UNAIDS Theme Groups, leaders of civil society organizations, NGOs, people living with HIV/AIDS, and donors to discuss the socioeconomic costs of the epidemic, examine best practices, propose specific solutions, and work to reach consensus on future activities. These meetings will be high profile and will be covered by the press. The teams will offer to work more intensively with governments that demonstrate commitment to developing a joint program of future activities. Celebrities such as football stars or musicians can also be engaged to appear on television and radio and at public rallies to mobilize civil society. The press will be heavily involved to raise the profile of these events.

- *Raise the issue in international forums.* International development organizations, including the Bank, should work to ensure that HIV/AIDS and its impact on development are top-priority agenda items at all high-level meetings involving Africa. These include the annual meetings of the Bank, the Southern Africa Development Community (SADC), the European Union, the East African Community, the G8, Club du Sahel, Comité Inter-Etats de Lutte Contre la Séchéresse dans le Sahel (CILSS), and the Organization for African Unity (OAU).

- *Develop country, subregional, and sector-specific presentations on the impact of HIV/AIDS on development, along with realistic solutions.* The president of the Bank, managing directors, regional vice presidents, executive directors, country directors, sector managers, and Bank staff from every sector frequently meet with their country counterparts in national governments. This provides an opportunity to raise awareness and develop innovative strategies for responding to the epidemic at all levels and in every sector. In Eastern and Southern Africa, there may be value added in initiating multicountry, subregional programs to curb the further spread of the epidemic. Subregional projects are being initiated by the Great Lakes and SADC countries. The Bank's AIDS Campaign Team for Africa (ACT*africa*) will work closely with UNAIDS and UNAIDS Theme Groups in countries to help develop these projects.

- *Sponsor and conduct conferences, workshops, and seminars to obtain broader buy-in for the intensified action.* The Bank will sponsor and participate in international and regional conferences on HIV/AIDS to strengthen partnerships with other organizations for this intensified action. In addition, ACT*africa* will conduct up to five workshops or seminars during fiscal year 2000, mainly in Africa, and offer future ones based on identified needs. These workshops and seminars may offer training to Bank staff and country counterparts on the socioeconomic costs of HIV/AIDS, the actual impact of the epidemic on development, design of programs, management and evaluation of HIV/AIDS projects, impact analysis, and projection modeling. Seminars will bring together technical specialists within and across sectors to brainstorm and develop innovative ideas for addressing the epidemic's impact within each sector.

- *Identify international and African firms to mobilize the private sector in Africa to join the efforts to intensify action.* International firms such as Levi Strauss and Shell Oil, as well as many national firms, are already incorporating AIDS-prevention activities into their workplace activities and can play an important role in mobilizing others in Africa. Enlisting the help of these firms, the Bank can organize meetings of business leaders throughout Africa to help them understand why they should take action and what they can do. Business interests as well as the social dimensions of their involvement will be analyzed further with the assistance of ACT*africa*.

1.b.   Build Local Capacity in National and Local Government, Civil Society, and the Private Sector to Lead and Implement Effective Programs

Governments and communities must take the lead to slow the spread of the epidemic and alleviate its impact on their societies. The capacity needed to respond is overwhelming and requires ongoing support and reinforcement. Not only is it necessary to expand knowledge and skills in controlling the epidemic, it is important to continually replenish the capacity as increasingly more professionals and skilled workers die of AIDS. Countries need to be planning ahead for the workforce needs that will result from the millions of premature deaths.

- *Provide technical assistance to countries.* The Bank is well placed to provide technical assistance to countries to assess the impact of the epidemic on the workforce and help sectors plan for replenishing the experience and skills lost. Technical assistance can also be provided to strengthen institutional capability to provide the multisectoral response that is needed.

- *Expand existing management training programs to include national leaders and staff dealing with the HIV/AIDS epidemic.* Managers at all levels involved in HIV/AIDS prevention and care need skills such as strategic planning, decisionmaking, and program, financial, and human resource management. By extending existing capacity-building programs that strengthen these general management skills to managers of HIV/AIDS-prevention and -care programs, the capacity to lead HIV/AIDS-prevention efforts will be increased. A needs assessment by countries and the Bank will determine which HIV/AIDS managers need skill development in these areas. Bank staff will work with country counterparts to plan and prioritize on the basis of identified needs.
- *Identify opportunities to modify existing Bank-financed projects and develop new projects to include strong components to build the capacity of people in all sectors to manage and implement HIV/AIDS-prevention and -care programs.* It is necessary to identify the training needs of people in all sectors to enable them to incorporate strategies to slow the epidemic and mitigate its impact. ACT*africa* will provide technical assistance to undertake these assessments. According to the assessed needs, Bank staff and country counterparts will incorporate training, study tours, and other capacity-building methods focusing specifically on HIV/AIDS prevention, care, and treatment.

2.   Strengthen the Bank's Own Capacity to Respond to Increased Demand

2.a.   Place HIV/AIDS as a Central Element of the World Bank's Development Agenda for SSA

Placing HIV/AIDS at the center of the Bank's development agenda for these countries and addressing it in all elements of the Comprehensive Development Framework will ensure that (1) innovative ways to slow the spread of HIV/AIDS and minimize its impact are considered within every sector and for every country with a growing epidemic; and (2) adequate resources are made available. Senior Bank management and country and sector teams will play a key role in integrating HIV/AIDS into the development agenda of the Bank and its country partners.

- *Provide resources and issue a clear statement (including instructions and timetables) from the Bank president and Africa regional vice presidents to country teams to address HIV/AIDS in all ongoing and future projects and activities in Africa.* The statement should challenge and support Bank staff to address HIV/AIDS in parallel with the Comprehensive Development Framework, looking for impact and identifying ways to reduce it. This will be done by providing funding to Bank country teams to assess, plan, and provide technical assistance. In addition, strong Bank participation will be required in UNAIDS Theme Groups in countries to strengthen the national response. This is especially important in countries where the Bank does not have a health portfolio. The Bank's active presence within the Theme Groups will demonstrate a corporate recognition of the relationship between HIV/AIDS and overall development. This will further the incorporation of HIV/AIDS into a country's larger development context.

- *Include HIV/AIDS as a required component of all country assistance strategies (CASs).* The Africa Region already incorporates HIV/AIDS prevalence rates in the table of key indicators of economic and human development appearing in each CAS, which defines the Bank's role in the future development of a country. But there is much more to be done. CASs for hard-hit countries should be expected to include credible plans, whether funded by the Bank or not, detailing how the country intends to address the epidemic. This will ensure that HIV/AIDS is part of the country dialogue. This not only raises the awareness of national leaders regarding the epidemic and its impact but ensures that the country program incorporates the necessary components to support a multisectoral, national program that is coordinated with UNAIDS and with donors.

- *Require AIDS impact assessments for all Bank projects.* Many Bank projects have the potential to either slow HIV/AIDS and mitigate its impact or contribute to further spread of the epidemic. An impact assessment is essential to decisionmaking and project design. The Bank can sharply improve analysis of the potential project impact on HIV/AIDS by screening projects for AIDS-prevention potential and recommending and financing the implementation of mitigation measures.

- *Issue a Bank operational policy (OP) or operational directive (OD) on HIV/AIDS.* The Bank will issue an OP or OD regarding HIV/AIDS to provide guidance to Bank staff on how to treat the issue in Bank policy dialogue and in Bank-financed projects and programs. It will provide guidance to countries to implement a policy framework that facilitates the use of tools known to be effective against HIV/AIDS. This would include, for example, laws that prohibit discrimination against people infected with HIV in employment or in access to health care. It would also provide mechanisms to allow people to be tested completely anonymously so that they can learn their status without risk that this information will be used against them. Both of these measures would encourage individuals to access VCT. An enabling policy environment would also include policies to subsidize purchase and distribution of condoms and diagnostic reagents.

2.b. Build Capacity within the Bank to Intensify Action against AIDS in Africa

To play a leadership role in mobilizing others to expand the response to the HIV/AIDS epidemic, the Bank needs to build the capacity of its own staff and provide the required tools and resources. Bank staff in all sectors need to realize the impact of HIV/AIDS on various sectors, and they will need country, subregional, and sector-specific data and projections to inform and influence their country counterparts as well as the tools and resources to incorporate them into projects. The data must be timely, accurate, and relative, yet easily understood by non-health professionals.

Demand for information and technical support is expected to increase once this strategy is approved. ACT*africa* has been established to meet this demand and support the mainstreaming of the HIV/AIDS agenda into all Bank activities.

- *Through ACT*africa, *provide operational support in mainstreaming HIV/AIDS activities in all sectors and actively promote intensified action.* ACT*africa* will serve as a critical resource to Bank task team leaders at the country, regional, and subregional levels. ACT*africa* will provide staff time of technical specialists who will support task team leaders in the design, implementation, and evaluation of projects with HIV/AIDS components in all sectors (see section 6 for detailed terms of reference). Seed money will also be provided to initiate HIV/AIDS-related activities either through ACT*africa* or directly to Bank country teams.
- *Expand operational support.* "Response agents" or team "affiliates" will be identified in resident missions and some Bank offices. These affiliates will be the responsible focal point in the country or sector to ensure implementation of the strategy and retrofitting of existing projects. These agents will be trained by ACT*africa* and will be extended members of ACT*africa*.
- *Develop tools and briefs for Bank country teams to inform and motivate their country counterparts to respond to the epidemic.* ACT*africa* will

develop tools for incorporating HIV/AIDS activities in all sectors. In close collaboration with UNAIDS, it will research, develop, and package country-specific HIV/AIDS status reports and presentations for all countries in the region and update them regularly. These tools will provide guidelines for task teams to assess needs and determine the most relevant actions to take.

- *Collect and disseminate information and documentation throughout the Bank and externally at central and country levels to inform staff and others of intervention tools and success stories.* ACT*africa* will collect information in close collaboration with UNAIDS. These documents will inform staff and can be further disseminated to country partners. ACT*africa* will also actively prepare information for the press and use the international press as a partner to inform and motivate others to take action.

- *Provide adequate resources to Bank country teams.* The work that has been done within the Bank in the past 14 months clearly demonstrates that country teams are willing to intensify HIV/AIDS activities in all sectors, given the resources. Additional funds will be earmarked for HIV/AIDS so that countries can carry out many of the activities proposed in this strategic plan. ACT*africa* will also provide technical support to the country and sector teams.

- *Develop and maintain Web pages to provide up-to-date information and best practices on HIV/AIDS and serve as a resource to Bank staff throughout the world.* Currently, the Bank operates two Web sites that deal with general HIV/AIDS issues and with the economic aspects of the epidemic. These need to be developed further, and additional ones established specifically for this initiative to serve as an efficient mechanism to disseminate valuable information. There is also a need to establish Web sites for the countries themselves to exchange experiences and lessons learned. These could be based on subregions (SADC, the Great Lakes region, West and Central Africa) or could be established for countries sharing a common language (French and English).

2.c. Strengthen Activities to Reduce the Impact of Socioeconomic Factors Influencing Epidemic Spread

Much of the work that the Bank and others are doing to reform health care, reduce poverty, improve the status of women, and build capacity are already helping to control the HIV/AIDS epidemic and mitigate its impact. Even though these programs do not specifically address HIV/AIDS, they address the root causes of vulnerability and deal with the very factors that allow the epidemic to spread. Therefore, it is important to continue supporting these strategies to help prevent further spread of the epidemic. There are few incremental costs associated with this objective, but the benefits are significant. ACT*africa* will work closely with the different networks, sector boards, and councils of the Bank to include HIV/AIDS activities in these areas.

- *Educate girls.* An increased level of education provides young girls with earning power to enhance their economic independence, which may keep them from resorting to commercial sex work for economic survival, thereby reducing their risk of HIV infection. Education also provides girls with the confidence and the basic knowledge to make sound decisions about their sexual health, again reducing their risk of contracting HIV. Increased efforts in girls' education are needed now because young girls are disproportionately infected and affected by this epidemic and by the many other reproductive health problems they face, such as female genital mutilation and unwanted pregnancy. Not only are they being infected with HIV, they are being pulled out of school to care for sick relatives or assume family responsibilities as their parents die. Efforts to increase girls' education should take these problems into account and find solutions to them.
- *Reduce poverty.* Poverty is an important determinant in this epidemic, forcing people to migrate away from their families to find employment or into commercial sex work for economic survival, placing them at high risk of HIV infection. The epidemic is also increasing poverty for families as resources that otherwise would have been spent on education fees, food, cash crops, or other productive investments are allocated to medical care for those infected. However, because poor households are more vulnerable to the impact of an AIDS death, general antipoverty policies and programs can also mitigate the impact of AIDS (World Bank, 1997a). The Bank must assist governments to create and maintain social safety nets, especially for families who have lost members to AIDS. ACT*africa* will collaborate closely with the Bank's ongoing poverty alleviation efforts.
- *Make health sector reform more HIV/AIDS-sensitive.* Health sector reform is predicated on reallocation of expenditures from non-cost-effective, predominantly curative interventions to those that are the most cost-effective, preventive, and community-based. Health reform is driven by legal, regulatory, and financial measures to

achieve decentralization, increased access, sustainable financing, individual responsibility for one's own behavior, and provider responsibility for service quality and coverage. All these elements are *also* crucial to creating an enabling environment to respond effectively to HIV/AIDS. Moreover, both health sector reform and HIV/AIDS challenge the current organization and management of the health sector (personnel, infrastructure, provider-client-community interaction); the health sector's ability to coordinate with other sectors/ministries; and the capacity to address both *biological* and *societal* vulnerability risk factors for disease.

Yet as the HIV/AIDS epidemic continues to grow, it increases the obstacles to health sector reform, which is needed now more than ever to ensure that health care is accessible to all. The costs of screening blood, HIV counseling and testing, drugs for STIs and opportunistic infections, and basic palliative care for AIDS patients are high, requiring more efficiency and financing alternatives. Through health sector reform, HIV/AIDS programs are being decentralized to districts without much-needed strong central guidance and sufficient resources. Those involved in health sector reform in countries that have very high HIV/AIDS prevalence need to consider the impact of this epidemic on the health sector in order to reach their goals.

- *Expand gender initiatives.* The HIV/AIDS epidemic has brought the effects of gender inequality to the forefront. Important strides have been made to improve the status of women and their role in society; however, much work remains to be done to enable women to make decisions that protect them from HIV infection, provide them with alternative means of protection, and afford them the economic freedom needed to survive. ACT*africa* will integrate relevant components of this strategic plan with Bank gender initiatives.

- *Improve reproductive health.* Africa possesses the world's highest maternal mortality ratio, highest infant mortality rate, highest fertility rate, highest unmet need for family planning, lowest contraceptive prevalence rate, and highest regional prevalence of HIV and other STIs. In addition to facilitating HIV transmission, STIs and their sequelae entail enormous health and socioeconomic costs, including infertility, congenital infection, and low birthweight. High fertility and rapid population growth impede efforts to reduce poverty, putting increased pressure on public funds so that there are fewer resources to invest in education, health, and other vital sectors. Strengthening and expanding existing reproductive health programs and integrating HIV/AIDS-prevention strategies will improve services and reach a large number of vulnerable women who are not being reached through other mechanisms.

- *Strengthen capacity building.* African nations will feel the impact of the HIV/AIDS epidemic for a long time to come and must be able to sustain their epidemic response to prevent further spread and mitigate the ongoing impact. Building the capacity of African governments, civil society (including NGOs and community-based organizations), and the private sector to mobilize and lead an effective response to this epidemic is critical. A long-term and sustainable response to the HIV/AIDS epidemic depends on building the critical mass of people in all sectors to replace those lost to the epidemic.

3. Expand Available Resources

3.a. Increase Funding for HIV/AIDS Prevention, Care, and Treatment

The Bank began funding HIV/AIDS-related projects in 1986. To date, it has committed over US$950 million for over 80 projects worldwide. Fifty-five percent of these resources are through the International Bank for Reconstruction and Development (IBRD) and 45 percent are through the International Development Association (IDA). Currently, there are three freestanding HIV/AIDS projects in SSA (Kenya, Uganda, and Zimbabwe) and a few more with HIV/AIDS components. The freestanding projects will be completed during the next 18 to 24 months, and no new freestanding projects are under preparation. An assessment needs to be conducted immediately to determine the consequences of either planning for follow-up projects or integrating HIV/AIDS components into health sector reform projects. Many countries, especially in Southern Africa, are reluctant to borrow and have relied on grant funding in the past. Given the gravity of the problem, the Bank should find a way to assist these countries through collaboration with bilateral or multilateral donors.

Many of the activities planned for this strategy will help reverse the decline in lending and grant support. Mobilization within the Bank and at the country level will increase demand among African governments for Bank resources for HIV/AIDS activities. Mobilization at the international level will increase grant resources from bilateral and multilateral donors.

- *Initiate and support Bank response.* In addition to the ACT*africa* core budget, country and sector directors will earmark money in their budgets specifically for HIV/AIDS activities. It is essential that funding comes directly from the country and sector budgets to provide task team leaders with the flexibility they require.

- *Provide grant support to the Bank.* Trust fund support of US$1 million from the Norwegian Royal Ministry for Foreign Affairs has enabled the current HIV/AIDS team to initiate several activities, including the preparation of this strategy. Additional grant funding will be required to sustain these activities for the next five years.

- *Provide Bank grant funding to UNAIDS.* The Bank provides a grant of US$3 million from its Development Grant Facility to UNAIDS to implement programs in West Africa, Southeast Asia, and Latin America and the Caribbean, and to provide core funding for the UNAIDS Secretariat. This grant must be continued to foster partnerships and support mobilization of resources at the national and regional levels, in addition to capacity building.

- *Redirect ongoing project funds to HIV/AIDS activities.* In many countries, ongoing projects can incorporate HIV/AIDS activities at little additional cost, simply by redirecting some funding toward HIV/AIDS activities or by redeploying some of the undisbursed resources already earmarked for HIV/AIDS activities. This will help to either scale up existing activities or start new ones.

- *Utilize innovative mechanisms to deliver resources to local governments, NGOs, and communities.* Social fund projects have been successful in channeling funds to communities by supporting NGOs, the private sector, and local governments. This strategy will take advantage of existing and new social funds to make resources available to communities. Modalities will be established to appraise and deliver funds to communities and NGOs through local governments, line ministries, implementing agencies, and/or regional NGOs, or directly to communities, civil society, and private sector organizations with proven management skills.

- *Include HIV/AIDS in the Heavily Indebted Poor Countries (HIPC) debt initiative.* An attempt will be made to include HIV/AIDS in the HIPC debt initiative promoted by the Bank. This existing mechanism may be used as an incentive to encourage countries to intensify their HIV/AIDS programs regardless of debt status and will be used to place HIV/AIDS prevention at the center of the country debt relief program and projects. Efforts will be made to integrate HIV/AIDS into reform programs, structures, and social policy reforms for beneficiary countries. The HIPC Trust Fund will finance HIV/AIDS activities through the national- or district-level AIDS programs.

3.b.   Use a Multisectoral Approach to Retrofit Existing Bank-Financed Projects to Reach More Vulnerable Populations and to Address Their Long-Term Needs Created by HIV/AIDS

This epidemic is seriously depleting valuable human resources in all sectors. Not only is it necessary to prevent further spread of infection, it is also essential to take steps now to alleviate many of the direct and indirect effects this epidemic will have on the sectors in the longer term.

Many ongoing projects in education, health and population, infrastructure, agriculture, and other sectors involve people who are vulnerable to contracting HIV. Integrating proven interventions against HIV/AIDS into ongoing projects would cost little, but it would greatly expand the number of people who hear the important messages and gain access to tools for prevention. People managing and implementing these projects need the encouragement and the tools to retrofit their projects with HIV/AIDS initiatives. The activities suggested below are just examples that can be applied in many different settings to expand coverage.

- *Assess the impact of HIV/AIDS on sectors and help countries plan for the long-term impact.* Funds will be provided to sector leaders and Bank country teams to support social assessment and impact studies and workshops to develop long-range plans. The Bank will provide technical assistance to countries to deal with the critical issues raised in this long-term planning for human resources and help countries analyze options.
- *Integrate HIV/AIDS education into existing school and training curricula.* Information about HIV/AIDS, how it is transmitted, and how it is prevented can easily be integrated into curricula for students at all levels; however, strong policies mandating this are needed to overcome the unfounded fears that this will increase sexual activity among youth. Opportunities for integrating HIV/AIDS education also exist at the college and university level, as well as in specialty training programs such as medical, nursing, architecture, agriculture, business, and trade schools. Governments can require that HIV/AIDS education be incorporated into all government training programs. Occupations that place people at high risk of infection should be particularly targeted with HIV/AIDS education. Particularly important are training programs for those working in transport/trucking, the military, and any occupation that makes people mobile and takes them away from their families for long periods. The cost of developing curricula and integrating them into existing

programs is minimal and can be done at the local level with little external assistance. Many ongoing and future Bank-funded programs in various sectors have education components that could be expanded to help prevent HIV/AIDS in these sectors.

- *Integrate HIV/AIDS education, condom distribution, STI treatment, and care and support into existing projects that employ workers who are vulnerable to HIV/AIDS.* Many Bank-funded projects employ people who are vulnerable to acquiring or transmitting HIV or are feeling the impact of HIV/AIDS on their family. These projects provide an opportunity to work with employers to provide the prevention, care, and support activities to their employees that will greatly expand the number of people reached. This goes beyond educating workers through brochures and training programs to (1) promoting condoms and making them available; (2) extending employee benefits programs to include treatment of STIs and opportunistic infections; and (3) extending these services to the families of workers. This same concept can be promoted to all employers in the Bank's work with the private sector. It is more than social responsibility; it will decrease the impact of the epidemic on all of these sectors.

3.c.   Mobilize the International Community to Leverage Additional Resources

Funding for HIV/AIDS in SSA has been declining, whereas the epidemic has been increasing over and above the worst projections. A new resource mobilization effort needs to be launched now to leverage additional resources from donor agencies and the private sector.

- *Take advantage of all major meetings the Bank attends with international partners, heads of state, and the private sector to raise awareness of the epidemic and its impact on development and to mobilize additional resources.* Bank senior management participate in many high-level meetings, such as the G8 and Bank annual meetings, and have an opportunity to influence their colleagues and leverage additional resources formally and informally through these meetings. The UNAIDS Secretariat will be organizing meetings for donors. Bank senior management can play an important role in these meetings, both in contacting donors and in lending its "weight" to such meetings.
- *Link with international donors to collaborate on or co-fund projects and research and to leverage additional funding.* Working in partnership with UNAIDS, other United Nations agencies, and international donors provides a much-needed synergism and results in less duplication of

efforts. Through jointly funded projects or research, the interventions or research applicability will reach a wider number of stakeholders and move toward reaching the scale necessary to slow the spread of the epidemic. In some cases, the Bank may have the technical expertise needed to complement funds provided by other donors, especially in countries reluctant to borrow.

- *Organize meetings of multinational companies to mobilize additional resources from the private sector.* Many multinational companies will be seriously affected by this epidemic, especially those depending on labor and resources from the countries hardest hit by HIV/AIDS. The Bank, in collaboration with UNAIDS, can organize companies that are already active in AIDS prevention as well as others to discuss the epidemic's impact and identify the important role they can play in this initiative.

- *Prepare briefing materials and presentation packages for Bank senior management to leverage additional funds.* In collaboration with UNAIDS, ACT*africa* will monitor the calendar of events for opportunities for senior management and executive directors to influence international partners and leverage resources at the central level. Country directors, resident representatives, and task team leaders will identify opportunities at the country level. ACT*africa* will develop generic and specific briefing packages to prepare Bank management to raise the issue of the severe impact of the HIV/AIDS epidemic on development. ACT*africa* will be available to meet with Bank senior managers and country teams to help prepare for each event.

4. Expand Available Knowledge and Develop Additional Prevention Tools

4.a. Identify Innovative Means of Financing the Development of Vaccines and Other Prevention Options, such as Microbicides

- *Develop new Bank instruments to strengthen the potential market for vaccines and microbicides and encourage the private sector to invest in more research to develop safe, effective, and affordable products for use in developing countries.* There is an urgent need for appropriate vaccines and other preventive tools that will be affordable, feasible, and effective in Africa. Currently, there is little effort to develop vaccines that will be effective against the HIV strains prevalent in SSA. To address this, the Bank has been working with the International AIDS Vaccine Initiative (IAVI) and established a Bank-wide AIDS Vaccine Task

Force in 1998 to examine means by which the development of an AIDS vaccine for developing countries could be accelerated. The AIDS Vaccine Task Force has consulted with numerous experts and sponsored studies of the pharmaceutical industry's perspective on HIV/AIDS vaccine research and development and of the potential demand for an AIDS vaccine in developing countries. It has also examined numerous institutional responses, including financial instruments that could be used to guarantee future markets for an AIDS vaccine in developing countries, which would encourage the private sector to invest. Another alternative is a financing infrastructure that facilitates the purchase of vaccines for poor countries once a vaccine or microbicide becomes available.

- *Promote female-controlled methods of prevention.* In Africa, women are at higher risk of HIV infection than men and have little power in negotiating condom use. Women in particular need alternatives to condoms that they can control and that will protect them from infection of HIV and other STIs. To date, research in this area is limited and more is needed to develop affordable alternatives such as microbicides. Mechanisms will then be needed to make sure they are widely accessible. Through its policy dialogue, the Bank can emphasize how female-controlled prevention options, such as microbicides and female condoms, must be complemented by more concerted efforts to address the underlying gender inequalities that impact women's risk of STIs and their ability to protect themselves with the existing range of prevention strategies.

4.b.   Support Research Efforts to Provide Decisionmakers with the Data and Tools Needed to Intensify Efforts

National leaders and international partners need accurate and basic information to make decisions on investing scarce resources in HIV/AIDS prevention and care.

- In collaboration with UNAIDS, fund and conduct studies on cost of treatment alternatives, cost-effectiveness, impact, cost of inaction, modeling of future impact and costs, and evaluate existing tools in different cultural and infrastructure settings. Experience has shown that leaders want to know how HIV/AIDS will affect their country's future development and what it will cost to respond. In addition, the cost of non-response can serve as a powerful motivating tool. Leaders in each sector will continue to view HIV/AIDS as a health issue unless they see the potential impact on their sector and the relatively low cost of intervention. Additionally, although much has been learned about what does and does not work in HIV/AIDS prevention, it is still necessary to evaluate the effectiveness of many of the existing tools in different cultural and infrastructure settings. The Bank will assess the need for research of this and other types at the regional, subregional, and national levels and will establish research priorities.

5

Planning for Implementation at the Country Level

This strategic plan has presented a rationale for immediate action and lists the concrete actions the Bank will take in collaboration with its partners to intensify action against HIV/AIDS in Africa. However, it falls short of describing how the Bank will work with countries to operationalize this strategy. Work is currently being conducted to provide a detailed set of operational guidelines and tools to help countries rapidly bring their HIV/AIDS-prevention and -care programs to a national scale.

Most current HIV/AIDS programs are implemented through government-run, vertical health sector programs or through small civil society organizations with limited funds and reach. Experience shows that, although many of the technical strategies used are effective, implementation cannot reach the necessary scale through these centrally operated programs. A decentralized, participatory approach involving all sectors will lead to wider coverage reaching all vulnerable people with appropriate interventions. The central government still has an important role to play in leadership, facilitation, co-financing, and coordination, thus creating the environment that will support an intensified and expanded response to the HIV/AIDS epidemic.

Translating operational guidelines into national, multisectoral programs with multiple partners will require strong coordination, practical toolkits describing best practices, coordinated procurement mechanisms, and complementary and flexible funding arrangements for all levels of intervention. Funding mechanisms will be identified that will quickly provide incremental and earmarked funds to the implementing agencies. The Bank will work with UNAIDS and other partners to quickly mount this coordinated response.

As these tools and mechanisms are being developed, ACT*africa*, with UNAIDS, will immediately begin identifying countries that have placed a high priority on scaling up their programs. ACT*africa* will review the portfolios of these countries to identify projects that can be retrofitted to strengthen HIV/AIDS-prevention efforts and will work with the Bank country teams to develop a detailed implementation plan that will list specific steps to be taken in all sectors to intensify efforts. ACT*africa* and UNAIDS will provide assistance and tools to accomplish the objectives established to expand and intensify efforts to prevent HIV/AIDS in the country.

6
Staffing and Support

This strategy document has clearly stated the need for the Bank to drastically increase its involvement in the fight against AIDS in Africa. ACT*africa*, which comprises a team leader, coordinator, broad-based economist, rural development specialist, technical specialist, four staff-year equivalents of short-term consultants, and two staff assistants, has been established to help fulfill this task. The team will also have "affiliated" members throughout the region who will devote a substantial amount of time to expand the capacity and sectoral expertise of the team. Most of ACT*africa*'s work will be demand-driven and funded from country budgets. The team will serve as the region's focal point and information clearinghouse on AIDS and will be responsible for the following major tasks:

- *Operational support to task team leaders in all sectors to mainstream HIV/AIDS interventions in their projects.* To expedite the mainstreaming of HIV/AIDS activities in the Bank's work, a Bank budget has been established to support initiation of these activities and enable ACT*africa* staff to focus on the development and implementation of these programs. This budget will be complemented with trust funds, which will be used to support the work of consultants and the organization of regional meetings and conferences. ACT*africa* will be responsible for the preparation of country briefs, good and bad practice notes, impact analyses, and other related outputs. ACT*africa* will also prepare public information materials, press releases, presentations, and background materials for use by Bank staff in advocacy and policy dialogue.
- *Development of tools.* ACT*africa*, in collaboration with UNAIDS, will prepare tools for project development and evaluation for both freestanding HIV/AIDS projects and those projects with HIV/AIDS-related components.
- *Contributions to CASs and policy dialogue.* ACT*africa* will provide analyses of the impact of the epidemic on various sectors and on overall development for use in CASs. These analyses will ensure that

HIV/AIDS is part of a country's development agenda and will provide task team leaders and countries with information critical to their long-term human resource planning. ACT*africa* will examine how HIV/AIDS is addressed in CASs and suggest improvements where needed. Additionally, ACT*africa* will assist Bank country teams with HIV/AIDS impact assessment requirements and monitor country programs to ensure that the needed actions are taken appropriately and in a timely fashion.

- *Knowledge management.* ACT*africa* will contribute to knowledge management by providing state-of-the-art information on all aspects of the epidemic within the Bank's knowledge management system, including HIV/AIDS Web sites. It will create much stronger links with the UNAIDS Secretariat and the World Health Organization (WHO) in the area of information compilation and dissemination.

- *Training, workshops, and networking.* The current strategy will be widely discussed in numerous national and international forums. The Bank's strategic plan will be presented at the 11th International Conference on AIDS and STDs in Africa, which will be held in Lusaka, Zambia, September 12–16, 1999, and the 13th International HIV/AIDS Conference to be held in Durban, South Africa, July 9–14, 2000. It was presented at the Fifth African–African American Summit in May 1999 in Accra, Ghana, and will be presented at the First International Conference on AIDS in Ethiopia, which will be held November 7–10, 1999, in Addis Ababa. Other regional meetings and workshops will be targeted to enable Bank staff in countries, the Bank's African counterparts, and other development partners to play a critical role in developing and implementing the strategy.

In collaboration with the World Bank Institute and other institutions, ACT*africa* will provide training to build broad capacity within the Bank to address HIV/AIDS in policy dialogue, projects, and programs. ACT*africa* will also conduct workshops for staff seeking to learn what is currently being done in their countries and sectors regarding HIV/AIDS and what interventions would be useful for them to apply in their work.

7
Next Steps

This strategy provides overarching guidance for the World Bank to intensi-fy its action against HIV/AIDS in Africa. It represents an initial and impor-tant step but does not provide the detailed guidance needed by country and sector teams to take many of the actions described in the strategy. ACT*africa* will begin immediately to work with Bank country teams and sectors to develop customized implementation plans and the tools essential to imple-mentation. Work is already in progress to determine the costs of scaling up HIV/AIDS programs to a national level for all countries in SSA. As previ-ously mentioned, a fully costed case study of an ideal program is presented in Annex 1.

References

AIDSCAP Project, Family Health International, The Francois-Xavier Bagnoud Center for Health & Human Rights of the Harvard School of Public Health and UNAIDS. 1997. *Final Report: The Status and Trends of the AIDS/STI Epidemics in Sub-Saharan Africa.*

Allen, S., A. Serufilira, J. Bogaerts, Van de Perre, and others. 1992. "Confidential HIV Testing and Condom Promotion in Africa: Impact on HIV and Gonorrhoea Rates." *Journal of the American Medical Association* 268 (23): 3338–43.

Bloom, David. 1998. *The Burden of AIDS in Africa.* Cambridge, MA: Harvard Institute for International Development.

Decosas, Josef, and Alix Adrien. 1999. Preliminary Discussion Draft. Background Paper on HIV Programming in Africa for the Canadian International Development Agency.

Decosas, Josef. 1996. "HIV and Development." *AIDS* 10 (supplement 3): s69-s74.

Gluck, Michael, and Eric Rosenthal. 1995. *The Effectiveness of AIDS Prevention Efforts.* Washington, D.C.: Office of Technology Assessment.

Grosskurth, H., F. Mosha, J. Todd, and others. 1995. "Impact of Improved Treatment of Sexually Transmitted Diseases on HIV Infection in Tanzania: Randomised Control Trial." *Lancet* 346: 530–36.

Jackson, D., J. Rakwar, and others. 1997. "Decreased Incidence of Sexually Transmitted Diseases among Trucking Company Workers in Kenya: Results of a Behavior Risk-Reduction Programme." *AIDS* 11: 903-909.

Kumaranayake, L., and C. Watts. 1999. *Costs of Scaling HIV Program Activities to a National Level for Sub-Saharan Africa: Issues and Methods.* Draft in preparation for World Bank.

Laga, M., A. Manoka, M. Kivuvu, B. Malele, M. Tuliza, N. Nzila, J. Groeman, F. Behets, J. Groeman, M. St. Louis, and P. Piot. 1994. "Condom Promotion, Sexually Transmitted Diseases Treatment, and Declining Incidence of HIV-1 Infection in Female Zairian Sex Workers." *Lancet* 344 (8917): 246-48.

Mann, Jonathan, and Daniel Tarantola, eds. 1996. *AIDS in the World II.* New York: Oxford University Press.

National Centre in HIV Epidemiology and Clinical Research. 1997. *HIV/AIDS and Related Diseases in Australia.* Annual Surveillance Report.

The Policy Project. 1999. *The Economic Impact of AIDS* (Draft). The Futures Group International.

Roberts, M., and B. Rau. 1997. "African Workplace Profiles." *Private Sector AIDS Policy.* Arlington, VA: AIDSCAP.

Rojanapithayakorn, Wiwat, and Robert Hanenberg. 1996. "The 100% Condom Program in Thailand." *AIDS* 10 (1): 1-7.

Swiss Federal Office of Public Health, AIDS Section. 1999. *HIV and AIDS National Program, 1999–2003.* Bern, Switzerland, February.

Topouzis, Daphne. 1998. *The Implications of HIV/AIDS for Rural Development Policy and Programming: Focus on Sub-Saharan Africa.* Sustainable Development Department, Food and Agriculture Organization, Rome.

UNAIDS. 1999a. *Prevention of HIV Transmission from Mother to Child: Strategic Options.* Geneva, May.

_____. 1999b. "Early Data from Mother-to-Child Transmission Study in Africa Finds Shortest Effective Regimen Ever." Press release. Geneva, February.

_____. 1998a. *Report on the Global HIV/AIDS Epidemic.* Geneva, June.

_____. 1998b. "World AIDS Campaign with Youth People." Press release. Geneva, April 22.

_____. 1998c. *Draft Report on Health Reform and HIV Workshop.* Geneva, June 24–26.

_____. 1998d. "New Initiative to Reduce HIV Transmission from Mother to Child in Low-income Countries." Press release. Geneva, June 29.

_____. 1998e. *AIDS Epidemic Update.* Geneva, December.

_____. 1998f. *Access to Drugs.* UNAIDS Technical Update. Geneva, October.

_____. 1997a. *Report on the Global HIV/AIDS Epidemic.* Geneva.

_____. 1997b. *Tuberculosis and AIDS.* Geneva.

United States Agency for International Development (USAID). 1997. *Children on the Brink: Strategies to Support Children Isolated by AIDS.* Arlington, VA.

United States Bureau of the Census, Population Division, International Programs Center, Health Studies Branch. 1998. *HIV/AIDS Surveillance Database.* Washington, D.C.

Wawer, M.J., N.K. Sewankambo, D. Serwadda, T. Quinn, and others. 1999. "Control of Sexually Transmitted Diseases for AIDS Prevention in Uganda: A Randomised Community Trial." *Lancet* 353: 525-536.

World Bank. 1999. *Population and the World Bank: Adapting to Change.* Washington, D.C.

_____. 1997a. *Confronting AIDS: Public Priorities in a Global Epidemic.* New York: Oxford University Press.

_____. 1997b. *Sector Strategy: Health, Nutrition, and Population.* The Human Development Network. Washington, D.C.

_____. 1993. *World Development Report 1993. Investing in Health.* New York: Oxford University Press.

Annex 1
Case Study

Planning a Multisectoral Program at the Country Level

Countries have been planning and implementing HIV/AIDS-control programs since 1985, and the process and product have evolved over time. In 1985, WHO began helping countries develop short- and medium-term plans for AIDS prevention and control describing the major strategies that government and donor agencies would support. These plans were coordinated by AIDS Control Program Managers based in the ministries of health. As the epidemic evolved, countries began to develop HIV/AIDS strategic frameworks and strategic plans with assistance from UNAIDS. These documents describe priority areas and activities based on the determinants of the epidemic in the country, but they rarely address the issue of sufficiently scaling up the program to halt the spread of the epidemic. Furthermore, the documents do not adequately address the issue of impact mitigation. As national plans evolved, countries began to involve leaders from other sectors in their strategies; however, the programs remained in the health ministries in most countries, and the approach is far from multisectoral in practice. Also, these plans rarely help sectors focus on the development impact of the epidemic and do not focus on maintaining adequate capacity or planning for staff turnover.

Prioritizing Key Components of a National HIV/AIDS-Prevention and -Control Program

There are many proven interventions that work synergistically to help people reduce their risk of HIV infection and prevent further spread of the epidemic. All of these interventions are in place at some level in most African countries, but they are not reaching enough people to slow the spread of disease, especially in those countries hit hardest.

It is critical to set priorities, choosing interventions that are most effective, address the most prevalent mode of transmission, and are sustainable. Depending on the stage of the epidemic, it is important to target interventions to those whose behavior places them at highest risk while increasing prevention efforts to reach all who are vulnerable. Although preventing HIV infection must remain as the highest priority for all countries, those with high or rising HIV prevalence must also begin to build the response for care, treatment, and support for those infected and affected by HIV.

HIV/AIDS-prevention messages must be appropriately targeted and constantly and consistently reinforced, and prevention tools and services must be affordable and easily accessible to all who need them. Interventions that are sporadic, reaching only a few, or that are not consistently available will not change social norms and will not slow the epidemic. A substantial amount of internal and external funding is needed to bring these interventions to a national scale, reaching all vulnerable people and sustaining the interventions until the epidemic is under control.

Operationalizing an Intensified Response

African governments that are committed to building their existing programs into an intensified and expanded multisectoral response must take the following steps to move forward:

- Declare HIV/AIDS a national crisis and immediately appoint a high-level national task force to assess the current status of the HIV/AIDS program, identify barriers and needs, and review the current national plan for HIV/AIDS to identify gaps. The task force would be composed of sectoral ministries, religious and cultural leaders, civil society, people living with HIV/AIDS, women's groups, youth groups, NGOs, CBOs, the private sector, and so forth. The task force, in conjunction with UNAIDS Theme Groups, should report to the highest level of government on the necessary actions to build an intensified national response and specify the resources needed.
- Gather data to forecast the impact of the epidemic on the country and specific sectors to mobilize leaders at all levels.
- Ensure that the body responsible for oversight and implementation of the national HIV/AIDS program has the power and resources needed to implement a true multisectoral response.
- Identify and mobilize critical partners.
- Appoint skilled and dedicated leaders to guide and manage the response.
- Mobilize the needed resources from the government budget, donor agencies, and the private sector.

- Build capacity throughout the country to respond.
- Mobilize communities to design and implement programs.
- Continually monitor and evaluate efforts and revise strategies appropriately.
- Join with other countries to benefit from subregional or regional activities and learn from others.

The case study provided below illustrates what can be done at the national level to halt the spread of the epidemic and minimize its impact. The comprehensive program described in the case study represents an ideal situation at which countries should aim. The success of the program will depend on commitment and resources.

Case Study: An Intensified National HIV/AIDS Program for Muzumbuka

The following case study is presented to illustrate what can be done at a national level to prevent HIV/AIDS and mitigate its impact. This hypothetical country is named Muzumbuka; however, this case study is based on a real country in Africa with moderately high HIV/AIDS prevalence that urgently needs to focus on prevention, care, and impact mitigation. Since no country in Africa is currently intervening in all the required areas nor at the scale required, this case study has been created to demonstrate the comprehensive response and scale that are needed to curb the epidemic. Cost estimates are also presented. The general principle of the interventions and the costing will be useful in planning similar programs in other countries.

In presenting this case study, it is assumed that Muzumbuka has a commitment to HIV/AIDS control at the highest level of government; is able to create an enabling environment, overcoming political and cultural obstacles; and has the absorptive capacity to intensify its efforts and bring the multisectoral epidemic response to a national scale. Each sector will also assess the impact of epidemic spread so it can plan to care for those infected and affected within their sector and fill the vacuum of skilled and experienced workers created by the epidemic.

Current Situation

Muzumbuka is an African country of 34 million people that serves as a major transportation hub for the East African region. Twenty-four percent of the population is urban and 47 percent of the total population is less than

15 years old. Muzumbuka borders countries that have been dealing with the HIV/AIDS epidemic since the early 1980s and was in fact one of the first countries to establish a national AIDS-control program. However, until recently Muzumbuka did not have a strong government commitment to HIV/AIDS initiatives, although the country had attracted multilateral and bilateral donor funds for HIV/AIDS.

In Muzumbuka, transmission of HIV occurs mainly through heterosexual contact beginning in the early teen years. Since 1983, when the first AIDS cases were reported, the HIV/AIDS epidemic has progressed differently in various population groups. Early in the epidemic, urban populations and communities along highways were most affected. In 1993, more than 60 percent of sex workers outside of major urban areas and 22 percent of truck drivers were HIV-positive. The rates of infection have continued to rise in populations practicing high-risk behaviors, such as sex workers, truck drivers, and the military, and now the epidemic has rapidly spread to rural communities. At the end of 1997, it was estimated that 9.3 percent of the adult population and 68,000 children were living with HIV/AIDS. Currently, there are over 520,000 orphans living in Muzumbuka. It is estimated that more than one million AIDS cases have occurred since the beginning of the epidemic, and approximately 940,000 people have died.

It is estimated that, because of AIDS, life expectancy will fall from 56 to 47 years by 2000 and that by 2010 the mean age of the labor force will decline from 31.5 to 29 years. This younger workforce will have less education, training, and experience.

Hospital data in Muzumbuka indicate that up to 50 percent of beds are occupied by patients with HIV/AIDS-related illnesses. Consequently, the demand for care and hospital supplies is enormous.

A National AIDS Committee (NAC) oversees the program in Muzumbuka and comprises representatives from several sectors. It is supported by the National AIDS Control Program (NACP) Secretariat. Both of these bodies are within the Ministry of Health (MOH). Although the annual budget for the national program is US$4 million, only 20 percent of this amount was actually mobilized over the last year. The NAC has not been effective in providing leadership because it has not made AIDS a high priority. The NACP is powerless because of the lack of financial and technical resources.

A 1995 situation analysis of HIV/AIDS in Muzumbuka demonstrated a lack of strong political will and commitment on the part of the government. Consequently, HIV/AIDS policy and sensitization activities at all levels were inadequate. Most people in the country, including key policymakers, still considered HIV/AIDS to be a health issue; thus, the multisectoral response was minimal. Weak government leadership had not promoted the appropriate individual, community, or national responses. Funding and other resources for HIV/AIDS activities largely depended on external resources, and efforts to curb the epidemic would have ceased if such funding had been cut off.

Implementing an Intensified HIV/AIDS-Prevention and -Control Program: What Needs to Be Done?

In 1998, the government of Muzumbuka changed. When the new government came to power, the NACP and the UNAIDS Theme Group presented national leaders with data illustrating the development consequences of the HIV/AIDS epidemic in the absence of an intensified, nationwide, and multisectoral effort. Subsequently, the new government declared HIV/AIDS a national crisis, committed itself to make the HIV/AIDS epidemic a national priority, and appointed a high-level national HIV/AIDS Task Force composed of sectoral ministries, religious and cultural leaders, civil society, people living with HIV/AIDS, women's groups, youth groups, NGOs, CBOs, the private sector, and others. In 1999, the Task Force, in conjunction with the UNAIDS Theme Group, intensified the national program to prevent further epidemic spread, care for those infected and affected by HIV/AIDS, and mitigate the impact of the epidemic on various sectors. The Task Force will expand the program over the next 5 to 10 years to reach 100 percent of the people at risk throughout the country. The Task Force will work in partnership with local governments, NGOs, the private sector, religious and cultural leaders, people living with HIV/AIDS, and bilateral and multilateral donor agencies. Specifically, the Task Force will do the following:

- The Task Force, with the UNAIDS Theme Group, will place its highest priority on prevention and will target interventions to those whose behaviors place them at higher risk of HIV infection. At the same time, the Task Force will scale up the program to reach women and in- and out-of-school youth—groups particularly vulnerable to HIV/AIDS. The interventions will also be scaled up to reach more people in rural areas.
- The highest priority will be reducing sexual transmission of HIV through STI management, condom availability, and behavior-change communication to discourage risk-prone behaviors. Although a lower percentage of HIV is transmitted through blood and from mother to child, interventions to prevent transmission via these routes will also be included.

- Assisting the country to care for, treat, and support the many ill and dying people will be a growing priority. Muzumbuka will strengthen communities' ability to provide the needed care, both through institution building and financial support. This community-based care must relieve some of the burden on the hospitals.
- Drugs will be procured and made accessible to all who need them to treat STIs and the opportunistic infections associated with HIV/AIDS, including tuberculosis. Antiretroviral (ARV) drugs will not be included in the strategy at this time because they are simply not affordable; however, the strategy will change based on new advances such as development and accessibility of other affordable, low-cost drugs. Muzumbuka will begin to strengthen the infrastructure needed to procure and deliver future drugs and new treatment possibilities.
- Religious leaders throughout the country have already joined together and pledged their support to the government in this effort. They have recognized the seriousness of the epidemic and have committed to revising their teachings and increasing their support to their constituents to help cope with the impact of the epidemic. Religious organizations will increase their role in counseling and community-based care. Religious leaders will continue to urge youth to delay their initial sexual encounter and encourage all to remain faithful to their partners; however, they will support the use of condoms for those who are not able to do this. Cultural leaders and elders in Muzumbuka are also committed to slowing the epidemic and have agreed to support major cultural movements to eradicate harmful traditional practices, including female genital mutilation, wife inheritance, and early marriage.
- Many NGOs in Muzumbuka are already active in HIV/AIDS-prevention activities, but their efforts have often been sporadic and lacked government support. Under the national Task Force, the NGOs have formed a coalition that not only coordinates efforts and shares resources, but also plays a strong advocacy role with the government.
- The Task Force has reached out to the private sector to join in the national response to HIV/AIDS by demonstrating the impact of the epidemic on their businesses. Business leaders have committed to integrating prevention and care activities into their existing programs, and some have already provided in-kind services such as public service announcements and advice on media development.

Creating an Enabling Environment

Program management. The NAC and NACP will be reorganized, made multisectoral, and moved above the level of MOH. The current staffing of both bodies will be assessed and revised based on skills and the need to represent multiple sectors. Clear roles and responsibilities will be developed. The UNAIDS Theme Group will coordinate all activities of the seven cosponsors and the bilateral and multilateral donors to ensure adequate and sustainable support to the intensified action plan.

Advocacy. The Task Force, with the Theme Group, will immediately collect data and develop tools to make presentations to leaders throughout Muzumbuka to mobilize additional support. This advocacy effort will address government, community, private sector, and religious leaders throughout the country and will invite them to join both the advocacy and response initiatives.

Policy development. The Task Force, with the Theme Group, will review and revise existing policies and develop new policies where needed to protect the blood supply, facilitate condom distribution by subsidizing costs, ensure adequate supply and accessibility of drugs for STIs and opportunistic infections, require reproductive health education in schools, ensure nondiscrimination and human rights, and address the issue of care for orphans.

Assessing impact and planning for the future. Each sector will assess the current and projected impact of the HIV/AIDS epidemic to determine how it can best respond to slow the epidemic among its workers; avoid contributing to epidemic spread; and plan for future resource shortages that will be created by the epidemic. Studies will examine how this epidemic will affect human resources, productivity, profits, and the manner of doing business. Once these facts are known, sector leaders will use the data to plan for future needs.

Program development and donor coordination. The Task Force will involve stakeholders in program development to ensure commitment. The Theme Group will establish a Donor Council to work closely with the reorganized NAC and NACP to ensure donor coordination and increase support.

Institutional strengthening. Although government, the Theme Group, communities, and the private sector at all levels will be involved in controlling this epidemic, many do not have the capacity to respond now. This low capacity will dwindle even further as the epidemic takes its toll. Institutional-strengthening programs will provide training and management systems and address the developing human resource needs. The Public Service Commission, with line ministries, has been asked to prepare a report for the Cabinet on the current response to HIV/AIDS, the impact of the epidemic on each sector, and what needs to be done. This report will inform the Cabinet on how to plan for human capacity for Muzumbuka.

Surveillance of HIV/AIDS/STI cases and behaviors. Sentinel surveillance programs are the most cost-effective way to monitor trends over time and ensure comparability of data. Muzumbuka will strengthen its current HIV/AIDS/STI surveillance program and initiate a program to monitor behavior trends through behavioral surveillance.

Monitoring and evaluation. The Task Force will establish indicators to monitor and evaluate its program. It will use the HIV/AIDS/STI sentinel surveillance and reporting data to monitor the epidemic trends. The Task Force will also use existing data sources such as the Demographic and Health Surveys to monitor behavior changes in the population.

Sectoral Activities

The Task Force will assist each sector to assess the impact of the epidemic and develop plans for integrating some of the prevention activities described below into its programs. The following sectors have already initiated plans:

Ministry of Youth (MOY). The government of Muzumbuka has placed special emphasis on protecting the next generation from HIV infection. The MOY will implement programs to reach all youth, in and out of school, with HIV/AIDS-prevention programs. This ministry will use popular sports figures and entertainment stars to lead campaigns specifically designed to help youth delay their sexual debut and adopt safe behaviors when they do become sexually active."Youth-friendly" health clinics will be established to offer youth reproductive health services and provide them with the tools to protect themselves.

Ministry of Education (MOE). The MOE will implement a policy requiring a reproductive health module to be developed and incorporated into all education programs, beginning at the primary school level. The first year of this program will be spent developing curricula on HIV/AIDS and reproductive health, printing materials, and training teachers to use these curricula. The additional costs for these activities will be nominal. Special mechanisms will be established to provide incentives for girls to remain in school longer. The MOE will also develop a mechanism to waive school fees for families that cannot afford primary education.

Ministry of Agriculture (MOA). The MOA will immediately train all agricultural extension workers in HIV/AIDS prevention and provide them with condoms for distribution and with information on where to access care and treatment. MOA officials will meet with the farmers' unions to identify further methods of preventing epidemic spread within their communities and to discuss the projected impact on their sector.

Ministry of Economic Development and Planning. The Public Service Commission, in conjunction with this ministry, has initiated data analysis and is developing projection models that it will use to plan for future resource needs in each sector.

Ministry of Finance (MOF). The MOF has initiated cost studies and developed models to determine the cost of this program. On the basis of these estimates, it will develop a budget for the government and a plan for leveraging additional resources from donor agencies and private sector partners. This ministry, with the support of international donors, has set up a social fund at the district level to enable families and communities to cope.

Prevention of HIV/AIDS and STIs

Behavior-change communication. Multiple media channels will be used to reach those at highest risk of infection as well as the general public to help people identify and change risky behaviors. The communication program will include mass media such as radio, television, and newspapers, as well as smaller-scale/personal outlets such as local drama, brochures and posters, counseling, school curricula, peer education, and workplace programs in all local languages. The interventions currently in place will be intensified to a national scale. They will go beyond raising awareness and increasing knowledge and focus on changing behaviors. Many of the training, school curricula, and peer education activities will be integrated into existing programs at little added cost.

Workplace intervention. The workplace offers a venue to efficiently reach large numbers of vulnerable people with HIV/AIDS interventions. All sectors, including the private sector, will help slow the spread of the epidemic and minimize its impact. This is particularly important when people's work places them at high risk for HIV. Interventions will include the behavior-change communication tools described above as well as condom distribution, treatment of STIs, and care for infected workers and their families. These interventions will also benefit surrounding communities.

Voluntary counseling and testing (VCT). Studies have shown that voluntary HIV testing with counseling is highly effective in changing people's behavior to reduce their risk both of being infected and of infecting others. In Muzumbuka, as in many other countries, counseling and testing services are inadequate. The challenge is to strengthen counseling and testing centers, create demand for these services, and provide them on a sustainable basis, making them available to all who want them. Lessons from other countries indicate that people are afraid of being tested, do not want to know their test results, and are concerned about confidentiality, resulting in low demand for these services. Strong policies will be implemented to protect the rights of people regarding privacy and test results. Muzumbuka will train additional counselors and expand its current pilot counseling and testing sites nationwide.

Management of STIs. Management of STIs is an important mechanism to control the spread of HIV for two reasons: 1) the presence of other STIs facilitates the transmission of HIV; and 2) diagnosing and treating STI patients provides an opportunity to counsel them about their high-risk behavior and provide them with condoms. A comprehensive STI management program includes communication to teach people how to recognize STI symptoms and where to seek treatment, as well as how to reduce the risk of contracting HIV. It provides timely and accurate diagnosis of STIs, appropriate treatment for the patient and his or her sexual contacts, and condoms. The government will develop and disseminate guidelines for syndromic management of STIs as well as strengthen the essential drug program.

Integrating STI treatment and counseling into family planning and maternal and child health services will also be explored. This integration would permit sexually active women to be reached with critical messages and treatment, which is especially important given the limitations of the syndromic approach for women.

Condom supply and logistics. The proper and consistent use of condoms is a highly effective means to prevent transmission of HIV and other STIs. Once people have learned the important role that condoms play in prevention and how to use them, it is critical to make them affordable and accessible to all. Condoms will be widely distributed at subsidized prices through social marketing, commercially through the private sector, and free through government programs. Muzumbuka will utilize these mechanisms to complement one another and expand the reach to different groups nationwide.

Blood safety. Though ensuring the safety of blood for transfusion is one of the most effective and easy-to-implement interventions, it is difficult to sustain blood-safety programs because of costs, logistics, and competing priorities. A comprehensive blood-safety program includes increasing the number of voluntary blood donors as opposed to paid donors, screening all blood for HIV and other infectious agents, and ensuring an adequate blood supply by decreasing the number of unnecessary transfusions. Muzumbuka will strengthen and expand its existing blood-safety initiative nationwide to include all of these components.

Reducing mother-to-child transmission of HIV. The vast majority of seropositive children acquire the virus as a result of mother-to-child transmission (MTCT), which can occur during pregnancy, delivery, or breastfeeding. Recent research advances have led to the development of a relatively inexpensive and logistically feasible ARV drug regimen for developing countries that reduces the risk of MTCT by 37 percent (UNAIDS, 1999b). This protocol involves having HIV-positive women begin an ARV regimen at the time of delivery in addition to a one-week postpartum regimen for both the woman and her newborn. This intervention remains dependent upon access to VCT and adequate infrastructure to procure and administer ARV drugs. Muzumbuka will build this infrastructure and plan for implementation of this regimen to reduce MTCT. It will gradually implement this program, beginning with a pilot project in selected urban sites. The government will also organize meetings to develop guidelines on other options for reducing MTCT, such as breastfeeding alternatives and vitamin A treatment.

Interventions for Care and Mitigation

Over 1.4 million people in Muzumbuka are currently living with HIV; nearly all of them will become ill and die within the next 10 years. All of these people will require health care and psychosocial support. Many will place a significant burden on their families, and many will leave orphaned children or elderly parents without support.

Strategies for caring for and supporting the vast numbers of people who are infected or affected by HIV/AIDS are few. The needs are already great in Muzumbuka, stretching the limits that primary, secondary, and tertiary health care levels can handle.

As families become devastated and fragmented by HIV/AIDS, communities in Muzumbuka must be prepared to take over, as the health systems simply cannot provide the care needed. Communities are willing to take on this responsibility but need the know-how, tools, and financial resources. The following strategies for caring for and supporting AIDS victims will be improved and brought to a scale that can cope with the growing epidemic.

Drugs to control opportunistic infections associated with AIDS. Low-cost drugs to control the common opportunistic infections associated with AIDS and to alleviate suffering will be a priority for Muzumbuka. These drugs will be procured and integrated into logistics systems to ensure availability to all who need them. Many of these drugs are already on the essential drug list but are often not available or affordable. The MOH will review essential drug lists to ensure that appropriate drugs are available, and logistics systems will be strengthened to increase accessibility.

Treatment of HIV/AIDS. The cost of the ARV drug regimens is prohibitive for Muzumbuka, as it is for most countries in Africa, especially when drugs for palliative care to treat opportunistic infections and reduce suffering are not available. The ARV drugs are expensive, and they require patients to follow a complicated, strict daily regime of medication, with frequent contact with health care providers. Muzumbuka does not have the health infrastructure to administer these drugs successfully nor to perform the complex tests needed for follow-up. At this time, Muzumbuka will work with UNAIDS and other countries in the subregion to evaluate treatment options and costs.

Home-based care. A person can be ill with AIDS for several years, making it a chronic illness requiring long-term care. Long-term hospital care for AIDS is not affordable nor even possible in Muzumbuka. Alternatives to traditional medical care will be examined. Some families with healthy care providers can take care of their infected family members at home but need the essential skills, tools, and financial resources to do so. The Task Force will assist communities to provide support services to build the skills, reduce the stigma attached to HIV/AIDS, and provide the most basic supplies such as gloves and disinfectants.

Hospice and hospital care. Hospitals are already overburdened with AIDS patients, doctors and nurses have not been adequately trained to care for them, and sufficient supplies and drugs are not available. Muzumbuka will continue to train health care workers in the treatment and care of AIDS patients and provide the needed supplies and drugs. It will also identify and strengthen other care alternatives.

Care for orphans and vulnerable children. Though extended families have traditionally cared for orphans in Africa, these extended families are being decimated and can no longer bear the full burden. Communities in Muzumbuka are meeting with the Task Force to determine how to bear this burden of caring for orphaned children. This goes beyond the basic needs of food and shelter to ensure their basic education and health care to decrease their risks of becoming poor and infected.

Psychosocial support. AIDS is not only a terminal disease that carries long-term physical suffering; its victims are often stigmatized. The physical and emotional suffering is immense. Little has been done to alleviate this suffering, and the existing social safety nets are simply not capable of dealing with these needs at the level required. As more people are affected by this epidemic, the psychosocial support needs increase. Yet the support networks are insufficient. Training for counselors and income-generation activities to support those infected and affected by HIV/AIDS are just a few of the interventions that Muzumbuka will develop to provide the support needed.

Projected Costs

Muzumbuka has conducted preliminary costing studies to determine a range of costs of selected interventions based on the size of the population covered (see Table A). The costing model used here calculates the size of the beneficiary group using available population, epidemiological, and

Table A. *Projected Annual Costs of Select Interventions*

Intervention	Implementing Agency	Projected Annual Cost in US$ Millions			
		100% urban coverage	25% urban coverage	100% rural coverage	25% rural coverage
Mass-media program	Ministry of Communication (MOC), Ministry of Information (MOI), Ministry of Education (MOE)	1	0.5	6	1.5
Workplace programs	Private sector and all government sectors	7	0.2	6.7	4
Voluntary counseling and testing	Ministry of Health (MOH), NGOs	4	1	10	3
STI management through STI clinics and integrated into reproductive health services	MOH, private sector	0.3	0.1	0.2	0.1
Condom social marketing	NGOs	20	4	37	9
Blood safety	MOH	0.6	0.2	2	0.5
Short-term ARV treatment to reduce MTCT	MOH	11	2.8		
Care of opportunistic infections and palliative treatment	MOH, CBOs, NGOs	24	6	26	6
Home-based care for AIDS patients	MOH, Ministry of Social Affairs (MOSA), CBOs, NGOs	7	2	7	2
Support for orphans	MOH, MOSA, CBOs, NGOs	216	60	227	60
Psychosocial support and counseling	MOH, MOSA, CBOs, NGOs	0.3	0.08	0.3	0.08

Note: These figures are based on a medium-cost scenario and are only used to demonstrate the differences in cost of certain interventions and coverage scenarios.

demographic information. Unit cost data for SSA were then taken from the literature and scaled up, allowing for varying cost structures and coverage scenarios. In general, the costs reflect only financial costs and represent the costs to scale up an existing program. They are presented as annual cost estimates in U.S. dollars for the year 2000 (Kumaranayake and Watts, 1999).

Despite Muzumbuka's intensified response to HIV/AIDS, the enormous resources required to scale up interventions to the national level will pose a challenge. Considering the resources available, the absorptive capacity, and the time required to engage all sectors, certain priority interventions have been chosen by the Task Force for the first year. Most of these key interventions are already in place at some level in Muzumbuka. All are not at a national scale, though the majority of these interventions have the potential to be scaled up relatively quickly. The Task Force has decided on the following priorities for the first year: a 100 percent awareness program, in both urban and rural areas; 100 percent VCT in urban areas and 50 percent in rural areas; 100 percent STI management in urban and rural areas; 100 percent condom social marketing in urban areas and 25 percent in rural areas; and 100 percent blood safety in urban and rural areas. The resource needs will range from US$20—US$49 million (see Table A).

The Donor Council that has been working closely with the Task Force and the UNAIDS Theme Group has managed to raise the necessary funding for the first year and firm pledges for the coming four years. The government of Muzumbuka is responsible for a significant portion of the budget.

Annex 2
HIV/AIDS Prevalence Rates
for SSA

Adult (15–49 Years) HIV/AIDS Prevalence Rates, Sub-Saharan Africa,
December 1997

Rank	Country	Adult HIV/AIDS rate (percent)	Rank	Country	Adult HIV/AIDS rate (percent)
1	Zimbabwe	25.84	23	Democratic Republic of Congo	4.35
2	Botswana	25.10	24	Gabon	4.25
3	Namibia	19.94	25	Nigeria	4.12
4	Zambia	19.07	26	Liberia	3.65
5	Swaziland	18.50	27	Eritrea	3.17
6	Malawi	14.92	28	Sierra Leone	3.17
7	Mozambique	14.17	29	Chad	2.72
8	South Africa	12.91	30	Ghana	2.38
9	Rwanda	12.75	31	Guinea-Bissau	2.25
10	Kenya	11.64	32	Gambia, The	2.24
11	Central African Republic	10.77	33	Angola	2.12
12	Djibouti	10.30	34	Guinea	2.09
13	Côte d'Ivoire	10.06	35	Benin	2.06
14	Uganda	9.51	36	Senegal	1.77
15	Tanzania	9.42	37	Mali	1.67
16	Ethiopia	9.31	38	Niger	1.45
17	Togo	8.52	39	Equatorial Guinea	1.21
18	Lesotho	8.35	40	Mauritania	0.52
19	Burundi	8.30	41	Somalia	0.25
20	Republic of Congo	7.78	42	Comoros	0.14
21	Burkina Faso	7.17	43	Madagascar	0.12
22	Cameroon	4.89	44	Mauritius	0.08

Note: Adult rates (percent) are derived from the number of adults (15–49 years) living with HIV/AIDS at the end of 1997 divided by the 1997 adult population. National HIV/AIDS prevalence rates are not know for the following four countries in SSA and consequently have not been included: Cape Verde, Sao Tome and Principe, Seychelles, and Sudan.
Source: UNAIDS, 1998a.

Annex 3
Annapolis Declaration

International Partnership Against HIV/AIDS in Africa

Meeting of the UNAIDS Cosponsoring Agencies and Secretariat
Annapolis, Maryland, 19–20 January 1999

Resolution to Create and Support the Partnership

Preamble

The HIV/AIDS situation in Africa has become catastrophic. The epidemic represents an unprecedented crisis for the continent. More than 20 million Africans are infected with HIV today. Over two million died of AIDS in 1998, including nearly half a million children. Four million new HIV infections occurred in Africa last year. In the most severely affected countries, a quarter of the adult population is infected. Hard-won gains in life expectancy and child survival are being wiped out. The AIDS-related suffering of individuals, families, and societies is enormous. Education and health systems are staggering under the burden as they lose trained professionals and incur higher costs because of the epidemic.

If left unchecked, the AIDS catastrophe in Africa will continue to worsen. The numbers of dead and dying will continue to grow exponentially.

The specter of such a huge tragedy calls for an emergency-style response from within and outside Africa. If such a response is mounted quickly, tens of millions of deaths can be averted.

Fortunately, a large-scale response is possible, to judge from recent encouraging signs of change. More national leaders are recognizing the seriousness of the situation and are speaking out, making AIDS a central development, social, and national security issue. There is evidence of successful national responses to HIV/AIDS in countries such as Uganda and Senegal, and of positive local responses within other countries. A number of international agencies are ready to increase significantly their commitment to fighting AIDS in Africa.

But current plans and actions are not enough. National awareness, commitment, and mobilization are still inadequate. Successes are too few and on too small a scale to reverse the epidemic. External support remains too small, slow and disjointed to have a critical impact.

In short, a much more substantial response to AIDS in Africa is needed urgently from all actors—governments, NGOs, local communities, the private sector, and international development organizations.

Resolution to Create the Partnership

In the light of this tragic situation, with AIDS fast becoming the number-one killer in Africa, wreaking even more havoc than civil strife and other diseases, the UNAIDS Cosponsors (UNICEF, UNDP, UNFPA, UNESCO, WHO, World Bank) and the UNAIDS Secretariat, meeting in Annapolis, Maryland, USA, on 19–20 January 1999:

- resolved to work together on an *emergency basis* to develop and put into practice an "International Partnership Against HIV/AIDS in Africa"
- urged all parties involved—and especially the primary actors, the African people and their governments—to act on an *emergency basis* to drastically slow the spread of HIV in Africa
- committed themselves to building rapidly a coalition of all the key actors: African governments; NGOs and other civil society organizations, including religious groups; bilateral and multilateral agencies; the private sector; and the UN system organizations
- agreed that a sustainable political and social mobilization on an unprecedented scale would be crucial for mounting an effective response to HIV/AIDS on the ground in Africa
- called upon the UNAIDS Secretariat to assume its responsibility to lead the further development and implementation of the Partnership.

Goals of the Partnership

The overarching goal of the Partnership is to urgently mobilize nations and civil societies to redirect national and international policies and resources so as to address the evolving HIV/AIDS epidemic and its many compelling implications. Only an urgent mobilization of this kind can curtail the spread of HIV, sharply reduce the impact of AIDS on human suffering, and halt any further reversal of human and social capital development in Africa.

The Partnership will pursue three major objectives through a series of actions that will be defined in conjunction with all the partners in the next few months. Notionally these include:

- *reduced HIV transmission,* as evidenced by declines in HIV incidence and prevalence in specific population groups, particularly in young people; by increased percentages of people with access to sexually transmitted disease (STD) treatment services; and by increased access of HIV-positive persons to mother-to-child transmission (MTCT) prevention services
- *reduced suffering,* as evidenced by an increase in access of HIV-infected persons to community-based care including, in particular, drugs for common opportunistic infections
- *mitigated impact of AIDS,* as evidenced by increasing numbers of countries with operational plans for mitigation, and an increasing percentage of families caring for AIDS orphans who are receiving special education, health, and nutritional services.

The Partnership will monitor the scale and speed of the response to the epidemic, including the number of countries implementing intensified AIDS programmes and the level of national and international spending on AIDS activities.

A small team from the UNAIDS Cosponsors will further develop a list of priority action areas before the end of February 1999, to be subsequently discussed and further refined with other partners.

Each African country will need to set its own national targets.

Main Values and Principles of the Partnership

It was agreed that members of the Partnership should embrace a set of common values and principles:

- strong African political leadership and commitment as the basis for effective action
- country focus and orientation to locally set priorities
- local institutions, including local governments, NGOs, and other community-based organizations, to be major actors
- participation of people living with HIV/AIDS
- openness to all persons and institutions prepared to join the Partnership and respect its values
- a sense of shared responsibility among all partners

- transparency of action and accountability for results
- respect for human rights and compassion for those suffering from HIV/AIDS
- willingness by U.N. and other external agencies to act flexibly and to complement one another on the basis of comparative advantage
- maximum reliance on existing organizational entities without the creation of additional bureaucratic structures.

Aims and Activities of the Partnership

Experience to date points to a number of "key elements" shared by successful national AIDS programmes and projects. The aim of the Partnership will be to support these elements of success on a large scale, so that successful responses to HIV/AIDS can be multiplied rapidly across all African countries.

The members of the Partnership will work to create a policy and social environment conducive to successful action (Attachment 1), by:

- developing strong commitment to confronting AIDS at the highest levels of government
- raising national awareness of the status of the epidemic and its devastating impacts
- fighting stigma and discrimination associated with HIV/AIDS
- empowering communities, NGOs, local governments, and the private sector
- inserting HIV/AIDS considerations more fully into the national development agenda
- protecting the rights of vulnerable populations
- organizing and implementing a multisectoral response
- harnessing external resources more effectively
- developing policies and plans that mitigate the impact of AIDS on key national sectors, institutions, and services, including education, health care, and agriculture
- raising the status of women

Within such a conducive policy environment, the members of the Partnerships will also support a series of priority programmatic actions, to be defined with the main partners over the next months. These will include a small sub-set of "core" actions necessary but not sufficient to be implemented in all countries. The core actions include: youth education and mobilization; voluntary counselling and testing; interventions to interrupt mother-to-child transmission; strengthening STD prevention and treatment; condom distribution; special programmes for those most vulnerable to HIV/AIDS; community standards of care, including treatment of common opportunistic infections of people living with HIV/AIDS; and special services for families with orphans. Programmatic actions should cover the reduction of both risk and vulnerability to HIV/AIDS.

While effective prevention activities must remain central to a national response—in both low- and high-prevalence countries—heavily affected countries today have an urgent need for policies and programmes that can soften the epidemic's *impact* on individuals and their families (especially the poor). They also need to anticipate and alleviate the effects on communities and productive sectors.

Main Lines of Action for the Partnership during 1999

To achieve its goals, the Cosponsors agreed that the Partnership will focus on the following main lines of action for 1999.

1. Mobilizing high-level African political support by discussing HIV/AIDS with African heads of state and striving to include AIDS in the central agendas of the Organization of African Unity (OAU), Economic Commission for Africa (ECA), Southern Africa Development Community (SADC), Economic Commission of West African States (ECOWAS), and so forth; developing and widely disseminating advocacy materials emphasizing the gravity of the AIDS crisis and its catastrophic demographic, social, and economic effects; and supporting the advocacy efforts of respected African figures from the political, cultural, religious, and sports spheres who seek to persuade African heads of state to commit themselves to attacking the AIDS crisis head-on.

2. Widening the partnership to include African governments and other key constituent groups including national and international NGOs, the business community, and bilateral and multilateral development institutions. As part of this effort, a donors' meeting will be held in the first half of 1999, possibly as early as March, and similar meetings will be organized for major NGOs and business partners.

3. Assisting African countries showing their commitment to the Partnership to design and implement intensified national AIDS programmes, by carrying out joint national/donor programme planning exercises in at least 10 priority countries over the next 12 months; mobilizing additional financial resources to support these intensified programmes through consultative group meetings and donor round-tables, incremental government financing (possibly linked to debt relief), and reallocating existing funds already committed to social funds and ongoing projects in the health, education, transport, labor, justice, and other sectors; and promoting active communication and information-sharing among all actors, including African communities and local governments, focusing particularly on examples of successful national and local initiatives.

4. Overall, mobilizing extra financial resources for intensified AIDS programmes at both country and regional levels. Current spending on AIDS in Africa, estimated at about $150 million a year, needs to be doubled to more than $300 million by the end of the year 2000.

5. Strengthening technical resources to support national and local projects, by:
- reviewing and rationalizing existing technical clusters located in the region, including the UNAIDS intercountry teams
- strengthening these technical groups through the hiring of additional key specialists
- building stronger networks of specialists in key programme fields (e.g., strategic planning, STD treatment, MTCT prevention, community mobilization, etc.) within and across countries.

Next Steps: Follow-on to the Annapolis Meeting

There are many actions that the UNAIDS Cosponsors and the Secretariat can take immediately, to drive forward the aims and activities of the Partnership. UNFPA, for example, will use its upcoming training programmes in Africa to expand AIDS activities in countries' reproductive health services. UNESCO will continue to implement its expanded network of community media addressing AIDS and to pursue research on cultural aspects of AIDS. WHO will drive home the messages of the Partnership with African political leaders and will strengthen its cadre of AIDS specialists in the region. UNDP will conduct a rapid assessment of its pilot projects on AIDS and Development, generate and disseminate best practice on HIV and development, strengthen the use of social capital in responding to the epidemic, organize stakeholder forums, and work with its resident coordinators in Africa on how to implement the goals and activities of the Partnership. UNICEF will step up implementation of its programmes for youth, AIDS orphans and the prevention of mother-to-child transmission.

The World Bank will build AIDS into the centre of all its Country Assistance Strategies, integrate AIDS into its agriculture extension projects, and reorient social fund projects to include local AIDS initiatives.

In addition, the Partners will pursue a common calendar of actions in the coming months, with all Cosponsors ready to take on extra tasks, many of them carried out jointly by several Cosponsors. The UNAIDS Secretariat will be responsible for overall monitoring of this plan of action. It will focus on political mobilization and on supporting the design and initiation of greatly intensified AIDS prevention, care and mitigation programmes in at least ten major countries before the end of 1999.

ANNAPOLIS, MARYLAND
20 JANUARY 1999

Attachment 1

Policy and Social Environment for an Effective Response to the AIDS Epidemic in Africa

Policy Area #1: Government Commitment

Objective: to achieve highest-level government commitment to confronting AIDS, as well as commitment in leadership groups at all levels, in order to mobilize for action, and to see this commitment reflected in increased allocation of national resources to HIV/AIDS.

Examples of instruments/actions:
- better advocacy based on reports on the status and impact of the epidemic
- development and use of compelling advocacy materials on best practice
- local advocacy groups, including people living with HIV and AIDS
- counsel from other leaders outside and in Africa
- AIDS on the agenda of regional political forums, such as OAU, ECA, SADC, ECOWAS

Policy Area #2: National Awareness

Objective: to raise national awareness of the status of the epidemic and its current and potential socioeconomic impact.

Examples of instruments/actions:
- generating and sharing experiences (good and bad practice)
- enhanced media partnerships, media training and support, community media
- improved surveillance of the epidemic, impact analysis, and dissemination of the findings
- laws on open, independent media.

Policy Area #3: Stigma and Discrimination

Objective: to fight the stigma and discrimination associated with HIV/AIDS.

Examples of instruments/actions:
- an effective ethical, legal, and human rights framework
- getting leaders, opinion-makers to speak out

- enabling people living with or affected by HIV/AIDS to speak out
- legal reforms and services against discrimination
- compliance with international treaties and statutes.

Policy Area #4: Local Empowerment
Objective: to empower local governments, the private sector, communities and NGOs to participate actively in designing and implementing parts of the national AIDS programme.

Examples of instruments/actions:
- legal and policy changes that permit easy creation and operation of NGOs and community-based organizations (registration, licensing, tax status, etc.)
- training of local government and NGO staff
- mapping and engagement of local groups
- alliance-building, networks of NGOs and local governments
- financing local groups via social fund mechanisms that encourage competitive, demand-driven design of local initiatives and cost-sharing
- work with local and international business associations.

Policy Area #5: National Development Agenda
Objective: to insert HIV/AIDS considerations more fully and prominently into the national development agenda, linked to poverty alleviation, better governance, debt reduction, etc.

Examples of instruments/actions:
- socioeconomic impact assessment
- agendas for consultative group meetings, donor round-tables
- debt-forgiveness as an incentive for increased national action, investment in HIV/AIDS.

Policy Area #6: Protection of Vulnerable Populations
Objective: to protect the rights of vulnerable populations, including children affected by HIV/AIDS (orphans, child-headed households, infected children).

Examples of instruments/actions:
- an effective ethical, legal, and human rights framework
- support (e.g., food and educational assistance) for families and com-

munities fostering AIDS-affected children
- legal reforms and services against discrimination
- compliance with international treaties and statutes.

Policy Area #7: Multisectoral Response

Objective: to implement a multisectoral response to the epidemic that includes centrally the health sector and institutions, but that goes well beyond health.

Examples of instruments/actions:
- creation of national AIDS commission
- multisectoral planning
- budgeting for multiple government agencies for HIV/AIDS.

Policy Area #8: External Resources

Objective: to harness external resources better and to increase the efficiency of planning for and implementation of externally financed HIV/AIDS activities.

Examples of instruments/actions:
- stronger UN Theme Groups on HIV/AIDS
- donor consortia using sector-wide approaches
- joint planning for national programmes.

Policy Area #9: Impact Mitigation

Objective: to support policies and programmes that reduce the negative socioeconomic impact of HIV/AIDS on production systems, public services, and households.

Examples of instruments/actions:
- programme development that anticipates and responds to losses of human resources in education and health systems
- programme design to meet the complex needs of children in AIDS-affected households
- teacher training and employment policies (e.g., use of paraprofessionals to supplement teachers) that take into account higher teacher morbidity/mortality from AIDS
- policies and projects for food security and rural development (e.g., pricing schemes and promotion of agricultural technologies better adapted to the needs of surviving spouses and elderly household heads)

- programmes to support the maintenance of capacity in key areas of public administration, including public utilities such as water and communications.

Policy Area #10: Status of Women
Objective: to strengthen the status of women in order to reduce their vulnerability to HIV and AIDS.

Examples of instruments/actions:
- legal reforms, legal services and counselling
- support to women's organizations
- support for changes in male sexual behaviour
- leadership development
- information and examples for informed debate
- girls' education.

Attachment 2

International Partnership against AIDS in Africa
Action Plan for 1999

1. Refine, finalize partnership concept and roadmap for action
   - revise and issue meeting statement   early February
   - develop and disseminate common "script" and description of Partnership   end February
   - intensify internal UN advocacy at senior level   February–April
   - discuss with Cosponsor country representatives   February–March
   - Partnership meeting to discuss framework agreement   April–May
   - public launch of the Partnership   September?

2. Mobilize political support
   - continue to seek input and endorsement of African leaders   February–April
   - support the efforts of the African leadership group   from March
   - develop advocacy plan and material   February–March
   - introduce into
     - –agendas of finance ministers (ECA)   April
     - –African health ministers (OAU)   May
     - –heads of state (OAU summit)   June–July

3. Engage donors, NGOs, and private sector
   - bilateral donors meeting   March
   - Partnership forum   April

4. Country-based programme intensification
   - UNAIDS Country Programme Advisors (CPA) retreat   January
   - UN Theme Group on HIV/AIDS (TG) to engage national political leadership and senior government counterparts   from February
   - country-focused impact/advocacy work   February–May
   - initial TG/national readiness assessments   February–March
   - intensified programmes under way in >10 countries   December

Annex 4
Strategic Options for the Prevention of MTCT

Prevention of HIV Transmission from Mother to Child: Strategic Options

UNAIDS—May 1999

Introduction

Mother-to-child transmission (MTCT) is by far the largest source of HIV infection in children below the age of 15 years. In countries where blood products are regularly screened and clean syringes and needles are widely available, it is virtually the only source in young children.

So far, the AIDS epidemic has claimed the lives of nearly 3 million children, and another 1 million are living with HIV today. Worldwide, one in ten of those who became newly infected in 1998 was a child. Though Africa accounts for only 10 percent of the world's population, to date around nine out of ten of all HIV-infected babies have been born in that region, largely as a consequence of high fertility rates combined with very high infection rates. In urban centres in southern Africa, for example, rates of HIV infection of 20 percent to 30 percent among pregnant women tested anonymously at antenatal clinics are common. And rates of 59 percent and even 70 percent have been recorded in parts of Zimbabwe, and 43 percent in Botswana.

However, there is no room for complacency elsewhere. African countries were among the earliest to be affected by HIV, and the epidemics on the sub-continent are therefore well advanced. But the virus is now spreading fast in other regions of the world, and everywhere the proportion of women among those infected is growing. Globally, there are about 12 million women of childbearing age who are HIV-positive. And the number of infants who acquire the virus from their mothers is rising rapidly in a number of places, notably India and South-East Asia.

The effects of the epidemic among young children are serious and far-reaching. AIDS threatens to reverse years of steady progress in child survival and has already doubled infant mortality in the worst affected countries. In Zimbabwe, for instance, infant mortality increased from 30 to 60 per 1000 between 1990 and 1996. And deaths among one- to five-year-olds, the age group in which the bulk of child AIDS deaths are concentrated, rose even more sharply—from 8 to 20 per 1000—in the same period.

The Risk of MTCT

The virus may be transmitted during pregnancy (mainly late), childbirth, or breastfeeding. In the absence of preventive measures, the risk of a baby acquiring the virus from an infected mother ranges from 15 percent to 25 percent in industrialised countries, and 25 percent to 35 percent in developing countries. The difference is due largely to feeding practices: breastfeeding is more common and usually practiced for a longer period in developing countries than in the industrialised world.

Prevention Strategies

Until recently, countries had only two main strategies for limiting the numbers of HIV-infected infants:

- primary prevention of MTCT—taking steps to protect women of childbearing age from becoming infected with HIV in the first place;
- the provision of family planning services, including pregnancy termination where this is legal, to enable women to avoid unwanted births.

These remain the most important strategies for reducing HIV among young children and essential activities in all national AIDS campaigns. Today, however, there is a third option for HIV-positive women who want to give birth which consists of a course of antiretroviral drugs for the mother (and sometimes the child), and replacement feeding for the infant. A recent trial in Thailand using a short course of zidovudine has shown that this strategy is able to reduce the risk of MTCT to below 10 percent when breastfeeding is strictly avoided. Alternative regimens using short courses of other antiretroviral drugs, sometimes in combination, will soon be available. Furthermore, trials are being conducted to find out what happens if mothers do subsequently breastfeed their babies instead of giving replacement feeds. This is a critical issue since the majority of HIV-positive women who risk transmitting the virus to their infants come from cultures where breastfeeding is the norm, and where replacement feeding presents great difficulties for many women.

Introducing a strategy of antiretroviral drug use and replacement feeding is, however, a complex process. To take advantage of the intervention, mothers need to know that they are HIV-positive, and they must therefore have access to voluntary counselling and testing. Costs and benefits need to be carefully assessed. Policy-makers need to decide what kind of programme is feasible and most appropriate for their countries, and whether or not to test models of the strategy in pilot projects before introducing it more widely. Such a programme requires a commitment to ensuring there is an efficiently functioning primary health care system with certain key services as a basis for introducing the strategy. Where these conditions do not already exist, decisions need to be made about how to strengthen the health infrastructure, what time-frame would be realistic, and what else is needed to create the conditions for safe and successful introduction of antiretroviral drugs and replacement feeding.

The purpose of this paper is to review the key issues for consideration in policy-making, and to propose ways in which the strategy might be tailored to suit local conditions. The paper is intended for all those with a part to play and a special interest in national policy making with respect to HIV prevention and care.

The Cost of Inaction

The cost of doing nothing to reduce MTCT will depend a great deal on the prevalence of HIV infection among parents-to-be. In areas where 20 percent or more of pregnant women are HIV-positive, the financial cost of caring for sick and dying HIV-infected children will be enormous, and there will be significant loss of the benefits from the huge commitment of time, energy and resources spent on reducing child morbidity and mortality over recent decades. Where HIV prevalence is low, health care costs will be relatively low too, and the waste of resources already spent on child survival not quite so dramatic. However, the costs for families and communities cannot be measured in financial terms alone, and many couples will bear responsibility for looking after their infected babies, often while struggling to cope with their own ill-health.

Major Issues for Decisionmaking

The following issues need consideration:

Counselling and voluntary testing

For women to take advantage of measures to reduce MTCT they will need to know and accept their HIV status. Voluntary counselling and testing services therefore need to be widely available and acceptable. Ideally, everyone should have access to such services since there are clear advantages to knowing one's serostatus. People who know they are HIV-infected are likely to be motivated to look after their health, perhaps with behaviour and lifestyle changes, and to seek early medical attention for problems. They can make informed decisions about sexual practices, childbearing, and infant feeding and take steps to protect partners who may still be uninfected. Those whose test results are negative can be counselled about how to protect themselves and their children from infection. Furthermore, voluntary counselling and testing has an important role to play in challenging denial of the epidemic: it helps societies which are currently only aware of people who are ill with AIDS to recognise that there are many more people living with HIV and who show no outward signs. However, it must be emphasized that, unless people have real choices for action once they have their test results, there is no good reason to take a test.

However, providing voluntary counselling and testing for the whole population will not necessarily be justified in low HIV-prevalence areas where resources are scarce. And even where justified on the basis of prevalence, it will not be a realistic option in some places because the health infrastructure is not sufficiently strong to support the service. For, besides the cost and practical requirements of providing counselling and testing itself, there must be an efficient referral system to a range of other basic services that people need once they have received their test results. These include family planning, prevention and treatment of sexually transmitted diseases (STDs), mother-and-child health services, and health care for infected people, including prevention and treatment of opportunistic infections, counselling, and psychological support.

Taking local conditions into account, therefore, policy-makers need to decide what kind of counselling and testing services are most appropriate and feasible, and what action, if any, is required to strengthen the health system that supports them. In particular, decisions need to be made about whether to make counselling and testing available to the whole population (comprehensive VCT); or to target the service at women or couples making use of reproductive health services in areas where the HIV prevalence is especially high (targeted antenatal VCT); or to offer counselling and testing to all women attending antenatal services as part of a programme to reduce MTCT of HIV (routine antenatal VCT).

Stigma and discrimination

Measures to reduce MTCT of HIV, especially the administration of anti-retroviral drugs and avoidance of breastfeeding, make it virtually impossible for HIV-positive women to keep their infection a secret from their families and people in the wider community. It is therefore essential to the safety and acceptability of MTCT interventions that effective steps be taken to combat rejection of people with HIV/AIDS. Where women fear discrimination, violence, and perhaps even murder if they are identified as HIV-infected, they will be reluctant or completely unable to take advantage of opportunities offered to protect their infants from infection. Special attention should be paid, in particular, to developing positive and non-judge-mental attitudes towards HIV/AIDS in health staff so that they can serve their clients with empathy. In places where stigmatisation of HIV-infected people is a serious problem, it would be advisable to introduce the anti-retroviral strategy for reducing MTCT in a pilot programme initially, so that the risks can be carefully monitored and ways of dealing with stigma and discrimination tested.

It is still common for women to be blamed for spreading STDs, including HIV, despite the fact that very often they are infected by the husband or partner to whom they are entirely faithful. To challenge this pervasive prejudice, as well as to encourage joint responsibility for childbearing and related decisions, it is a good idea to offer counselling and testing to pregnant women's partners also, where this is feasible and desired.

Health care systems

A programme of voluntary counselling and testing, antiretroviral drugs and replacement feeding can only be set up where there is an efficiently functioning health system with certain key services. Mother-and-child health services, including widely available and acceptable antenatal, delivery, and postnatal services, are essential. And counselling services, family planning services and medical care for HIV-positive women and their children should also be part of the basic health care provision. These services need to be carefully prepared for the integration of the new programme. In particular, steps are required to ensure:

(a) easy access and privacy for clients attending services. This will require assessment of the physical environment of clinics, and perhaps rearrangement of activities;

(b) continuity of care and a good flow of information between the various units involved in the management of HIV-positive clients;

(c) technical supervision of services to enhance quality;

(d) opportunities for clients to express their needs and their views.

Where the basic services are already in place and operating efficiently, the cost of providing counselling and testing, antiretroviral drugs and replacement feeding is likely to be well distributed across the health system and relatively easy to absorb. However, in places where the health infrastructure needs considerable strengthening and perhaps even building from scratch to support the new programme, the additional cost will assume greater significance. Since expansion and improvement of the health system benefit the whole of society, it is important that the MTCT programme is not expected to bear an undue and perhaps crippling proportion of the costs and responsibility. If the provision of antiretroviral drugs and replacement feeding is to be sustainable over the long term, the financial burden must be fairly distributed across the health services. Policy-makers should take account, also, of the fact that improvements in access and quality of services have a tendency to increase public expectations of health and therefore the demands on the health services.

Replacement feeding

The issue of replacement feeding is a complex one. Promotion of breast-feeding as the best possible nutrition for infants has been the cornerstone of child health and survival strategies for the past two decades and has played a major part in lowering infant mortality in many parts of the world. It remains the best option for the great majority of infants, and in providing for replacement feeding as part of the strategy to reduce MTCT of HIV, policy-makers need to take into account the risks of undermining breastfeeding generally, and of relaxing vital controls on the promotion of infant formula by the industry. They also need a sound assessment of how safe it is to recommend replacement feeding in their local setting. For example, is infant formula readily available; is the supply of formula assured over the long term; do people have access to clean water and fuel for boiling it; and are they sufficiently educated and informed to make up replacement feeds correctly? If used incorrectly—mixed with dirty, unboiled water, for example, or over-diluted—breastmilk substitutes can cause infection, malnutrition, and death. Where the risks associated with replacement feeding are not clear, research will be necessary to establish the facts, and strategies should be tested in pilot projects. The fact that the fertility lowering effects of breastfeeding will be inactivated makes the availability of family planning services as part of post-partum care a necessity.

Pilot Projects

In many places it will be a good idea to introduce prenatal voluntary counselling and testing and the use of antiretroviral drugs and replacement feeding in a limited way in pilot programmes initially, so that lessons can be learnt about how best to operate the new service before it is introduced more widely. Careful monitoring and evaluation of such an exercise are essential and must be planned for from the start. Pilot programmes are specially important in places where stigmatisation of people with HIV/AIDS is common, and where there is uncertainty about the safety of replacement feeding, or the acceptability of voluntary counselling and testing. Pilot sites should be selected on the basis of having good basic health services (as described above) already in place and efficient referral systems. Only if the projects are successful under these carefully chosen pilot conditions will further testing be tried in more challenging environments.

Integration of services is a key requirement: measures to prevent MTCT of HIV are one part of the wider programme to cope with HIV/AIDS in a country, and should have strong links to all other aspects of the programme, such as primary prevention of infection, care of infected people, and the support of orphans.

The Wider Benefits of the Package of Interventions

Providing voluntary counselling and testing, antiretroviral drugs and replacement feeding for the reduction of MTCT has benefits that extend way beyond the direct benefits to the health and survival of infants. All pregnant women, mothers, and infants will benefit from the expanded provision and improved quality of health care, especially mother-and-child health, antenatal, delivery and postnatal services. And the population as a whole will benefit from general strengthening of the health infrastructure, as well as from the increased understanding and acceptance of the HIV/AIDS epidemic and those affected that develop as a consequence of counseling and testing and measures to combat stigmatisation. A decision to introduce the package of interventions can, in the first place, be a force for social change, providing the opportunity and impetus needed to tackle often long-standing problems of inadequate services and oppressive attitudes.

Questions of Ethics

A guiding principle behind the introduction of any measure to reduce MTCT is that it is the pregnant woman's absolute right to choose, on the basis of full information, whether or not to take advantage of the intervention. Coercion is not justified under any circumstances, even if it seems to be in the best interests of the woman or her child, and her choice should always be accepted and respected.

Introducing antiretroviral drug programmes for the prevention of mother-to-child transmission in countries where antiretrovirals are not available for the treatment of HIV-positive people more generally has raised sometimes heated debate about the ethical implications. The question is asked: If a mother's access to antiretroviral drugs is limited to the period of pregnancy and labour, does this amount to treating the mother for the sake of her baby alone? In fact, the question is based on an erroneous perception, for an antiretroviral drug used for the purpose of preventing MTCT of HIV is not really a treatment, but a "vaccine" for the infant. A useful analogy is the rubella vaccine given to pregnant women to protect their offspring from the ill-effects of maternal infection. Rubella vaccination does not meet with ethical objections, despite the fact that it, too, could be seen as treating the mother for the sake of the baby.

The fact that antiretrovirals can serve two separate purposes—as vaccine for infants against MTCT of HIV, and as treatment for HIV-infected individuals—is, of course, very significant. But the issue of antiretroviral treatment for infected people must be considered separately from the issue of antiretroviral drugs used for the prevention of MTCT. It requires debate and policy decisions outside the scope of MTCT policy-making. However, it is a point of principle when adopting a strategy of antiretroviral drug use and replacement feeding that HIV-positive pregnant women must be assured of the best possible care available in their countries. In some places antiretroviral drugs will be available for therapy, too; in others, such treatment will simply not be feasible.

It is important also to note that a short course of antiretrovirals during pregnancy, while increasing the chance that she will give birth to an uninfected baby, does no harm to the health of an HIV-positive woman. The only possible risk is anaemia. But anyone taking antiretrovirals for HIV should be screened for this condition in advance, and treated for it if necessary. Concern is sometimes expressed that the strategy might encourage the development of drug-resistant strains of HIV. However, the risk of resistance developing is minimal with such a short period of drug use.

Another concern is the idea that introducing this strategy for the prevention of MTCT might exacerbate the problem of orphaned children, increasing the burden of care on families and society. It is widely assumed that infected infants do not survive long enough to become orphans. But this is a misconception: in fact, around half of such infants are still alive at their fifth birthdays and beyond and are highly likely to survive their infected mothers. The most likely effect of introducing the strategy, therefore, will be to alter the proportion of orphans who are HIV-infected compared with those who are uninfected.

For example, it is estimated that, of 100 infants born to HIV-positive mothers in the absence of intervention, roughly 66 will be uninfected, 17 will be infected and die before the age of five years, and 17 will be infected but still alive at their fifth birthdays. With the intervention, roughly 90 will be uninfected, five of the remaining ten who are infected will die rapidly and five will survive longer-term. Thus, with or without the intervention, more than 80 percent of the babies born to HIV-infected mothers will be exposed to the risk of being orphaned by the age of five years. The intervention does not therefore affect in any significant way the need for societies to make provision for their orphaned children. However, from the point of view of planning for care and allocating resources, it is important to recognise that, with measures to reduce MTCT, many fewer orphaned children will be HIV-infected and in need of medical care and support, many of them long-term. It is also worth noting that improving perinatal care and diagnosing HIV infection to permit early access to care may prolong the life of mothers. HIV-positive women may also live longer if they do not have to cope with sick children. Thus, their children will have the care of their mothers and be spared the misery and vulnerability of orphanhood for longer.

Affordability and Cost-effectiveness of the Strategy

The affordability of antiretroviral drugs and replacement feeding will depend a great deal on the condition of the health infrastructure within a country or district, and how much strengthening or expansion of services is needed before the strategy can be introduced.

Antiretroviral drugs for mothers known to be HIV-positive and replacement feeding for their infants is affordable in most countries, or districts within countries, where there are already well-functioning health care systems. For instance, countries that would be able to negotiate a price for the drugs of US$50 per woman, and infant formula at US$50 for six months, would need to spend US$130 per pregnant woman with HIV, including the costs of counselling and other inputs. In countries with a birth rate of 40 per thousand, and 15 percent HIV prevalence among pregnant women, and assuming that all women who know their status (estimated to be 10 percent) accept the intervention, the cost per capita of the specific inputs (i.e., drugs and replacement feeds) would amount to US$0.08. This calculation does not take into account savings of medical and other expenditures to care for HIV-positive infants—which, though admittedly very low in some countries, can be substantial in others. In fact, the savings may more than compensate for the cost of the intervention. Nor does it take into account the wider benefit of the intervention to the general population, which, as has been shown, is often considerable.

Voluntary counselling and testing also needs to be taken into consideration. If the cost of this service is to be borne exclusively by MTCT prevention programmes, the cost-effectiveness of the strategy will depend on the HIV prevalence in the area: the lower the prevalence, the more it will cost to identify each HIV-positive pregnant woman. Models show that cost-effectiveness remains fairly stable at HIV prevalence rates of 5 percent to 10 percent and over, but that where the prevalence rate is below this, the cost-effectiveness of the intervention rapidly decreases as the prevalence rate drops. In such situations, targeting HIV screening at women who are pregnant or who plan a pregnancy in specific population groups will lead to greater cost-effectiveness.

Cost-effectiveness by HIV Seroprevalence

Where HIV prevalence is high, the cost of a programme of voluntary counselling and testing, antiretroviral drugs and replacement feeding compares well with the cost of interventions for other health problems. It is estimated, for example, that at HIV prevalence rates of 5 percent and above, this strategy costs around US$35 per disability adjusted life year (DALY), compared with US$20–US$40 per DALY for polio and diphtheria vaccination, and US$200—US$400 per DALY for river blindness prevention.

Definition

Disability-adjusted life-years (DALY) are the number of years of life saved through a particular intervention, discounted slightly for each successive year saved to take account of the fact that the quality of life diminishes as time passes and the risk of dying of some other disease increases. Thus, the first year of life saved as the consequence of the intervention counts as a full year, whereas each successive year counts for a little less each time. The great strength of DALYs is that they reflect both quality of life and chances of survival and allow for easy comparison between different kinds of intervention.

A Decision Tree

Clearly, national and local circumstances will have a major influence on decisions regarding the adoption of voluntary counselling and testing, antiretroviral drugs, and replacement feeding. The following "decision tree" is proposed as a means of assisting those involved in national and local policy-making to decide on (a) the appropriate levels of provision, and (b) the best model of operation of the strategy.

The influencing factors:
- Seroprevalence of HIV in the country or community will determine the costs of inaction and the relative cost-effectiveness of different screening strategies.
- Attitudes towards HIV in the country or community will determine the risk of discrimination against women found to have HIV, the likelihood of infringement of their rights, and the expected acceptability of the intervention.
- The risks associated with replacement feeding will determine whether or not the intervention can be introduced on a large scale immediately or whether pilot projects will be needed initially so that lessons can be learnt about how to make replacement feeding safer.
- The state of the existing health system and mother-and-child health services (including family planning) will determine the expenditure of effort and resources required to strengthen them sufficiently to support the new programme.
- The maturity of the epidemic and level of social support that has developed to cope with it will determine how big a burden will be imposed upon the MTCT programmes by increased demand for health care and counselling.
- The wider benefits to society will have to be taken into account when balancing costs and benefits of the intervention.
- Available financing for MTCT interventions and associated services will be a major consideration in decisionmaking.

These factors will vary a great deal from one place to another. The following table proposes a decision-making process to assist policy-makers who wish to consider adopting an antiretroviral drug and replacement feeding strategy that is suited to their situation, and that reflects the local HIV prevalence, available resources, health system performance and expected risks associated with replacement feeding.

Definitions

1. Local health system meets requirements: Access to adequate mother-and-child health services including antenatal, delivery, postnatal and family planning services and continuing medical and psychosocial support for mother and child

2. Short ARV: Regimens as used in Thailand study, i.e.,
300 mg ZDV bid from 36 weeks
300 mg ZDV 3-hourly during labour
(Note: alternatives to the Thai regimen will soon be available for short ARV)

3. Long ARV: Other regimens including ACTG 076 and regimens using a combination of antiretroviral drugs and antiretrovirals for the neonate as well as the mother.

4. Known HIV-positive: Women who present for antenatal care having already been tested for HIV outside the maternal health services, and found to be infected.

5. Targeted antenatal VCT: Voluntary counselling and testing offered to pregnant women and their partners in communities (geographical or social networks) where HIV prevalence is particularly high.

6. Routine antenatal VCT: Voluntary counselling and testing offered to all women attending antenatal services and their partners as a matter of course

7. Pilot introduction of VCT and ARV/RF: Introduction of the full strategy in a selected number of sites, and careful monitoring and evaluation of the processes and their impact, with particular attention to replacement feeding

8. Prepare the health system: Where the health system does not meet the requirements for the successful introduction of the strategy, careful

preparation is needed for voluntary counselling and testing, mother-and-child health services, and medical and support services for seropositive women and their children.

List of Documents on MTCT Available through UNAIDS Information Centre or through UNAIDS Web Site (www.unaids.org)

General Information:
- UNAIDS Technical Update on HIV Transmission from Mother to Child (October 1998)
- Prevention of HIV Transmission from Mother to Child : Planning for Programme Implementation. Report from a Meeting, Geneva, 23–24 March 1998
- Prevention of HIV Transmission from Mother to Child: Strategic Options (May 1999)
- AIDS 5 years since ICPD: Emerging issues and challenges for women, young people and infants (1998)

HIV Counselling and Testing:
- Counselling and voluntary HIV testing for pregnant women in high HIV prevalence countries: Guidance for service providers (May 1999)
- The importance of simple/rapid assays in HIV testing. WHO/UNAIDS recommendations (WER 1998, 73, 321-328)

Antiretroviral Treatments:
- WHO/UNAIDS recommendations on the safe and effective use of short-course ZDV for prevention of mother-to-child transmission of HIV (WER 1998, 73,313-320)
- The use of antiretroviral drugs to reduce mother to child transmission of HIV (module 6). Nine guidance modules on antiretroviral treatments (UNAIDS/98.7)

HIV and Infant Feeding:
- HIV and infant feeding: A review of HIV transmission through breastfeeding (UNAIDS/98.5)
- HIV and infant feeding: Guidelines for decision-makers (UNAIDS/98.3)
- HIV and infant feeding: A guide for health care managers and supervisors (UNAIDS/98.4)
- WHO/UNAIDS/UNICEF Technical Consultation on HIV and Infant Feeding Implementation Guidelines. Report from a meeting, Geneva

20–22 April 1998
- HIV and infant feeding: A UNAIDS/ UNICEF/WHO policy statement (May 1997)

Planning, Implementation and Monitoring & Evaluation:
- Vertical Transmission of HIV—A Rapid Assessment Guide (1998)
- Local Monitoring and Evaluation of the Integrated Prevention of Mother to Child HIV Transmission in Low-income Countries (1999)

MTCT Prevention in Asia:
- Thaineua V. and others. From research to practice: Use of short-course zidovudine to prevent mother-to-child HIV transmission in the context of routine health care in Northern Thailand (*South East Asian Journal of Tropical Medicine and Public Health*, 1998).

MTCT Prevention in Latin America:
- Prevention of vertical transmission of HIV. Report from a workshop, Buenos Aires, 29–31 July 1998.

MTCT Prevention in Africa:
- The Zimbabwe Mother-to-Child HIV Transmission Prevention Project: Situation Analysis.